Cancer Relativity

A Unified Theory

Ray Reynolds

Plowboy Publishing Inc.

ISBN-13: 978-1515011989
ISBN-10: 1515011984

CONTENTS

Ray Reynolds

1 INTRODUCTION

"Just because physicians are smart, doesn't necessarily mean they have commonsense."

About a year ago while at my home in Thailand I noticed that a quarter inch diameter white lump had appeared on my forearm. It looked like one half of a Pearl glued to my skin. I went to the local hospital and showed it to their dermatologist who did a biopsy and determined that it was basal cell carcinoma, the most prevalent and least dangerous of all the skin cancers. His solution to the problem was to make an incision all the way around the tumor at a distance of 1 inch so that he would be sure to get all the root system. Obviously this sort of procedure would have left considerable disfigurement. I went on the Internet and started looking for an alternative to surgery.

What I discovered was that hundreds of people had successfully eliminated basal cell carcinomas by simply applying an ascorbic acid and water paste directly to the cancer and that within a week it would be dissolved with no scarring whatsoever. I decided to give it a try and after about four days the ascorbic acid had dissolved the quarter inch hemisphere of the carcinoma down to below skin level. I then watched with fascination as it traveled laterally just under my skin consuming the cancer cells as it followed the root system that had been established by the growth.

On my next visit to the dermatologist I showed him where the carcinoma had been and how well the skin was healing. He just smiled at me and said "Good job!" He knew about that kind of treatment, he knew that it would probably work but he couldn't recommend it to me because it was not an "Approved Procedure" within his medical peer group.

About three months later I had just completed a minor surgical procedure and was still under anesthesia in the recovery room when I suffered a myocardial infarction involving the coronary arteries that feed the lower apex of both ventricles. This resulted in 2 1/2 hours of CPR followed by a one-week coma. Over the next three months I slowly recovered heart function and was doing quite well until I suddenly went into congestive heart failure. I was admitted to Lee Memorial Hospital in Fort Myers Florida where I spent a week being treated for that condition. My heart function was so impaired that I could not walk more than 20 feet without stopping and gasping for breath. A healthy heart has an ejection fraction of 50% to 70%. Mine was less than 20%.

I began researching two things on the Internet, the first of course, was for any possible cure for my current condition. The other was a painless way to kill myself if recovery was not possible! I was very fortunate to find a copy of Dr. Stephen Sinatra's book the "Sinatra Solution" on Kindle. In it he explains the simple regime of supplements that he has used for the last 30 years to help his congestive heart failure patients. I had my wife bring the four main supplements to the hospital and began taking them about three days prior to my discharge. When I finally left the hospital and returned home I was not able to walk up the stairs to the second story without stopping halfway up to rest and gasp for breath.

Within one week of continuing to take the supplements I was able to run up the stairs two steps at a time for 10 repetitions. The main reason for this rapid recovery was that our heart cells have the remarkable capability of being able to go into hibernation when deprived of oxygen. This allows them to stay alive for as much as a month on the meager supply of oxygen that leaks past a coronary artery obstruction. After the blockage is removed and those heart cells once again are receiving oxygen they are often incapable of resuming normal function until they have also received sufficient nutrition to develop the energy resources to restart and continue their normal contractions.

The nutritional supplements that I was taking provided the high plasma concentrations needed to allow those stunted heart cells to revive and resume their normal contractile function. Now all of this begs the question, why the hell didn't my cardiologist tell me about those four critical supplements that had made such a miraculous difference? The answer, of course, is the same. The use of those supplements was not an "Acceptable Procedure" within his peer group of fellow cardiologists."

The bottom line is that if I had just gone along with what the professional medical personnel recommended and prescribed I would not be sitting at a computer writing this book! We must all learn to do our own research and educate ourselves about all of the possible solutions and then and logically analyze them for any value that they may have and then utilize it to our fullest advantage. I have completely recovered my cardiopulmonary function and am living in the high Sierra of Southern Peru where there is 17% less oxygen per breath. So obviously sometimes alternative treatments can be very effective.

Likewise there are many alternative cancer treatments, which seem to be equally effective but contradict each other. Some tell us that an acidic body PH is conducive to cancer growth and that we should avoid consuming berries because they are acidic. They ignore recent research that has proven berries to be the best source of anti-angiogenic factors, which prevent the growth of capillaries within cancer tumors thereby limiting their size to less than a dozen cells.

Others claim that consuming only protein and fat, which causes the body to switch from glucose to ketone usage for energy will cause cancer cells to starve to death because they can not use ketone sugar for energy production. Vegetarians take the other side of that argument insisting that too much fat and protein consumption will cause cancer. Once people have formulated a concept and convinced themselves that it is true they tend to become very resistant to change no mater how compelling new information may be. This is especially true of physicians and other professionals.

Perhaps a better approach would be to examine the different theories without prejudice with an eye to combining their best attributes in a logical manner creating a unified synergistic approach that has much greater efficacy than any single system by itself could provide.

For at least 20 years researchers have noticed a correlation between obesity and cancer. Because of this they assumed that fat caused cancer. Recent research however has proven that it is not the fat that causes cancer but rather the large amounts of sugar and high glycemic index foods people consume in order to produce the fat. Sugar in and of itself is a systemic inflammatory, which contributes both directly and indirectly to cancer and coronary disease. Also the process of converting blood glucose into fat for storage is highly inflammatory. It is not the fat in and of itself which causes a problem but the processing, storage and then utilization of the fat for energy that causes obese people to have a far greater risk of cancer.

It is easy for even experienced research biologists to assume that when two things occur simultaneously one of them is causing the other when in reality there is a hidden third factor in the equation that is causing both. This is just one of the many logic traps that we must be aware of if we are to succeed in sorting out the best combination of alternative treatments to achieve our goal of cancer prevention or cure.

Anti-carcinogenic nutrients are very synergistic. If consuming an ounce of strawberries or blueberries per day increases your cancer resistance by 10% it is very possible that consuming 1/2 ounce of each together will provide a 30% resistance. The same is true with green tea. Research studies have proven that combining two different varieties of green tea provides six times the cancer prevention of drinking one or the other by itself. This concept of "synergistic interaction" between various anti-carcinogens is very common so we need to determine which combinations of them are best for achieving maximum efficacy

We need to determine the commonalities between the different Cancer treatments that have proven effective. Is there something that they all advise doing that makes them mutually effective? Are they synergistic and complementary? Many alternative cancer treatments are very dogmatic and deviations from what they prescribe are not allowed. The problem with this is that some of the treatments which are equally successful contradict each other as well as contradicting recent cancer research.

Modern Western medicine is seriously bipolar. On the one hand we have the best medical technology available anywhere in the world. If you are involved in an accident and are suffering from severe traumatic injuries our emergency room services will save you if it is at all possible. On the other hand when it comes to treating chronic degenerative diseases such as cancer, obesity, high blood pressure and diabetes we seem to be a complete failure. The assumption seems to be that these diseases of modern lifestyle are first of all inevitable and secondly next to impossible to cure.

Since the turn of the 19th century our environment has become progressively polluted by chemicals and poisons. Our food supplies are grown in soil that has become hopelessly depleted of its trace minerals, which have been inadequately replaced by chemical fertilizers. The concept of crop rotation to help restore the balance of soil fertility seems to have become a lost art. Chronic drug use in the northern hemisphere has caused pharmaceutical pollution to the point where the penguins in Antarctica are pissing Prozac! Our drinking water has become so contaminated with drug residue that a glass of water from the kitchen faucet provides us with our daily allotment of prescription drugs whether we need them or not. As a result of this people's bodies have become progressively poisoned.

During the 1800s the death rate from cancer was less than 1 in 200. In 1900 less than 1 in 24 people were cancer victims. In the 1940's 1 in 16. In the 1970's 1 in 10. Today 1 in 2 men and 2 out of 3 women will suffer from cancer at some point in their lives. Clearly people who lived in the early 1800s were much healthier than we are today. This in spite of a lack of modern medical miracles such as vaccines, antibiotics and high blood pressure medications.

For the last 5000 years of recorded medical history all of the healthcare systems from Hippocrates to traditional Ayurvedic, Chinese, and Arabic medical practices have been based on nutrition and herbal supplements. Today physicians receive almost no training in the nutritional aspects of immune system support. And when a cancer patient asks their oncologist what they can do nutritionally to help their bodies cure their cancers they receive an evasive and ambiguous answer which amounts to "There's nothing you can do except take your medications." I have not been able to find any cancer textbook that oncologists use in their training that says a word about the role of nutrition for curing cancer.

There are several reasons for this, the primary one being the prohibition of any information by physicians that does not originate from what is referred to as "evidence-based medicine." This refers to the standard double-blind placebo-controlled human research studies that drug companies use to test their new medications. This is carried to such an extreme that oncologists ignore any evidence provided by studies performed on animals and only accept information based on large-scale human studies.

Until confirmation is provided by these human studies your typical oncologists either has never heard of a particular study or if he does happen to hear about it will simply ignore its results as being irrelevant or invalid. The cost of these human trials for a single medication can be anywhere from $500,000 to $1,000,000. Obviously if the study needs to be performed on a substance that cannot be patented and therefore no profit can be made from it that study will never be financed. This is the "Catch 22" of cancer research.

Rather than offering more complex and accurate advice concerning nutrition and health to laypeople who would require substantial education prior to being able to understand the nuances of proper nutrition physicians can more easily offer a pharmacological solution. On the other side of the coin the food industry does not want people to become aware of the link between processed foods, cancer, obesity and heart disease. These two powerful industries provide much financial incentive to all parties involved including the US government to not interfere with the status quo. On the other side of the problem are the population in general who are set in their dietary ways and do not want to change. They would just as soon opt for the simple solution of taking a pill.

Everyone fears cancer, it's only natural as it can appear suddenly with devastating results. The statistics clearly state that if heart failure doesn't kill you first then cancer will eventually. According to the FDA there is no cure for cancer only treatments. Fortunately there is much that we can do to prevent cancer and to treat it when it does occur.

Recent studies at the University of California at Berkeley have determined that cancer is not a genetic disorder but one in which healthy cells have been forced to alter their normal biology in order to deal with changes to their environment caused by the external influence of chemicals, radiation, stress or unhealthy diet. (Biochem J, 2000; 348: 497–506).

If after 100 years of research and $2 trillion of funding we are no closer to a cure for cancer I think it's about time that we reengineered the whole process. If we can't rely on the health care industry to prevent and cure cancer can we do the job ourselves? And if so what is the most effective combination of treatments both mainstream and alternative to accomplish that goal. Those are the questions I will try to answer in this book.

Ray Reynolds

2 THE DEMOGRAPHICS OF CANCER

For the same age groups the prevalence of breast, prostate and colon cancer are nine times greater in the United States and Europe than in Southeast Asia and the Orient. Breast cancer in particular is a disease of rich women. It is prevalent in Hong Kong where everyone is very wealthy but not on mainland China where there is almost universal poverty. The rate of cancer for the Japanese who have lived in the United States for most of their lives is almost the same as the average rate for persons born and raised in the US and whose genetics are 100% Western.

Apparently genetics is not much of a factor in cancer rates. More than 80% of cancers have external factors rather than genetics as their cause. Stomach cancer which was prevalent during the 1960s has almost completely disappeared in only 40 years. This has been attributed to the lessened use of nitrites for the preservation of food. Detoxification of the body has always been a main tenant of every major medical system for the last 3,000 years and it is even more important today than ever.

Since cancer is primarily an affliction of Western populations it would probably be a good idea to figure out what the differences are between our lifestyles here in America and Europe and the lifestyles in the Orient and Asia where cancers are nine times less likely to occur. Our human ancestors who lived more than 100,000 years ago were hunter gatherers and that lifestyle is still firmly imprinted within our genetics. The only sugar they had easy access to was from fruit which was seasonal and not continually available to them throughout the year. Also any fruit they might consume contained cancer fighting nutrients so it was probably more of a plus than a negative. They also ate no cereal products such as wheat or rice which today are the two most prevalent sources of carbohydrates other than sugar.

In evolutionary terms 100,000 years is nothing and our bodies and genetics still expect the same diet that was available back then before agriculture was ever invented. Today more than 50% of our caloric intake is derived from three sources that did not exist when our genetics were evolving. During Paleolithic times the annual consumption of sugar per person was less than 2 pounds but by the turn of the 21st century it had risen to more than 100 pounds per year. The second category of food that we consume the most of is white bleached flours that even most insects will not consume probably because they don't recognize it as a food source. The third major food group that makes up that 50% of the average American diet is vegetable oil.

These three food categories contain no essential vitamins and minerals or any of the nutrients needed to sustain our health. One thing that they do very well is directly contribute to the development of cancer. This website (http://globalcancermap.com) has an interactive map of the world where you can click on any country and determine what their rate of cancer is. One of the reasons that I currently live in southern Peru is that their cancer rate is 50% less than the United States and Europe. The cancer rate in Bolivia which is a much poorer country is 70% less than the United States and Europe. Clearly as far as cancer risk is concerned living in a pueblo in the Bolivian Andes is three times healthier than living in the developed countries of the world.

A complete imbalance in the ratios of fatty acids and the consumption of very high glycemic index foods are the defining characteristics of the Western diet. These are the same conditions which are very conducive to the growth of cancer cells in laboratory studies.

3 THE ECONOMICS OF CANCER

Today there are more people making a living from cancer than are dying from it. During their treatment cancer patients are lost in a maze of tests, second opinions, more tests and endless treatments in a system that feeds an immense medical apparatus that employs millions of people. When we add to that the medical schools, clinics and pharmacies it is obvious that the cancer treatment system has itself become a financial cancer that currently consumes $65 billion per year just to exist.

If a simple cure for cancer were discovered that entire $65 billion a year business of cancer treatment would be wiped out overnight. The science of cancer therapy is not nearly so complicated as its' politics and economics. If cancer patients are not benefiting from conventional cancer treatment they at least have the satisfaction of knowing that they are supporting the most profitable business in history.

The world pharmaceutical industry is without doubt the most profitable and least regulated business that has ever existed. In 1992 Congress passed the drug user fee act authorizing drug companies to pay user fees to the FDA for every drug that it submits to the FDA's approval process. Basically this act put the FDA on the payroll of the pharmaceuticals industries that it supposedly is in charge of regulating. The FDA currently receives half of its financial support from the pharmaceutical companies rather than from the US government. At the same time many of its 18 advisory committee experts who help to evaluate drug efficacy also work for the drug companies.

Pharmaceutical companies currently pay the FDA more than a half billion dollars annually most of which comes from the $1.4 million application fee that they pay the FDA for each drug that needs approval. This permit fee structure was not imposed by the US government but was actually requested by the drug companies who went to Congress to lobby for its' approval. This allowed them to do two things, they essentially purchased the FDA's drug evaluation department from the government, and at the same time eliminated competition from the smaller pharmaceutical startups who could not afford to pay the application fee for the approval of any medications they might develop. After the institution of this new fee structure the time required to approve a new treatment went from 24 to 6 months.

Roche one of the worlds largest pharmaceutical companies is a major beneficiary. Its two chemotherapy drugs, Avastin for colon cancer and Herceptin for breast cancer account for a large part of the company's 10% increase in year over year profits. In the US Avastin generates annual sales worth $2.3 billion. Avastin costs from $4,000 to $8,000 per month. Other chemotherapy drugs can cost as much as $10,000 per month.

Despite over $2 trillion having been spent in the war on cancer since 1970 we are no closer to a cure than we were 100 years ago. The aviation industry has gone from a wooden contraption that could barely fly a couple of feet off the ground to jet powered behemoths that transport hundreds of people across oceans in hours and are considered to be the safest form of transportation available. Communication has gone from simple telegraph to sophisticated satellite communication systems, cellphones and Internet. The difference is that these technologies make their money from improvements to their efficiency. Whereas the cancer treatment industry makes more money through inefficiency than it would if it actually developed a cure.

4 IT ISN'T EASY FOR PHYSICIANS EITHER

Throughout history the dominant theme of scientific discovery has centered around the complete rejection by the scientific community of any new theories or discoveries that contradicted currently established beliefs. Almost universally those scientists who proposed a new theory were denounced as quacks or charlatans. Columbus was ridiculed for claiming that the earth was round instead of flat. Galileo was imprisoned for claiming that the earth was not the center of the solar system. William Harvey was denounced by other physicians because of his research which demonstrated that the heart pumps blood throughout the body in a circular pattern. Even as late as the 1800s doctors who recommended that physicians wash their hands before operating on patients were ridiculed and often terminated from their teaching positions.

During French explorer Jacques Cartier's second voyage of exploration in Canada his ships become stuck in ice while transiting the Saint Lawrence River and his sailors began to die from scurvy. The Iroquois Indians told him to treat them using a tea made from the bark and needles of the white pine tree which is rich in vitamin C. His sailors after drinking the tea were immediately cured of their scurvy and when he returned to France he informed the medical establishment there of his discovery, which was immediately ridiculed and not followed up on. During the next 200 years from 1600 to 1800 more than a million sailors needlessly died from scurvy. Finally in 1747 John Land a young surgeon's mate in the British Navy suggested that lemons or oranges be included in the diet of British sailors to prevent scurvy but it was another 50 years before the British Navy's medical personnel implemented this practice.

Physicians are forced to practice what is called consensus medicine this means that they must not deviate from the practices utilized by their fellow physicians which are considered to be the norm. Innovation is not allowed unless it meets with the approval of the rest of the medical establishment. The only three procedures which are currently approved by the AMA and the FDA for the treatment of cancer are surgery, chemotherapy and radiation. They both assert that there are no cures for cancer only treatments. In a Harvard University study 85% of the oncologists they surveyed stated that neither they nor their families would ever undergo radiation or chemotherapy for cancer.

As a training exercise medical students are continually presented with patient symptoms in their classes and they and their professors then try to diagnose which medical problems could cause them. This deductive process can require as much as thirty minutes to accomplish. Obviously in the real world by that time the patient will have died. An experienced physician upon being presented with a patient who is symptomatic can usually diagnose what is causing the problem within 30 seconds. If you ask him what parameters influenced his decision he probably will not be able to tell you. His decision was influenced not only by the sounds he heard through his stethoscope but also the subconscious input from his other senses as well.

Physicians routinely make mistakes in their diagnosis and treatment of patients, it's endemic to the process. The third leading cause of death after heart disease and cancer is medical error. Quite often diagnosis of a patient's problem becomes a process of elimination through examination and testing. Usually any attribution errors are not fatal and once the proper diagnosis is arrived at the patient is treated and sent on his way. Misdiagnoses are rather common in emergency room situations especially when the patient is unconscious or otherwise incapable of describing his symptoms.

The attending physician usually has no knowledge of the patients medical history and must rely on strictly empirical evidence and symptoms which can often be similar for different ailments. This is compounded by the fact that the triage nurse in a busy emergency room may assign three separate cases within 30 minutes to a particular doctor who then has to sift through the foggy memories of the patients for historical clues to determine if the problem was pre-existing. If not, he then tries to find out from the patient or his immediate family what may have occurred in the patient's life just prior to his experiencing the symptoms. All of this can cause the physician to render a diagnose too rapidly and treat them for a condition they did not really have.

What physicians need to do is think outside the box beyond the immediate possibility and consider other often times rarer complications that could be causing the patient's symptoms. Insurance companies and HMOs unfortunately try to limit a physicians patient examination time to fifteen minutes or less. Physicians tend to shy away from the diagnosis of a rare disease favoring instead more common disorders which have most of the same symptoms. This works very well 90% of the time. But if you happen to be one of the 10% that is suffering from an uncommon illness it definitely works against you.

It is often quite expensive to do the specialized testing for a rare disorder and health insurers and HMOs are very reluctant to pay for what they consider unnecessary testing. Another reason why unusual disorders are seldom diagnosed correctly is that most doctors have no personal experience with them. If the problem is being caused by a nutritional deficiency the odds of a correct diagnosis are very low as physicians receive very little training in the symptoms of poor nutrition.

Sometimes physicians will subconsciously eliminate a couple of minor symptoms which fall outside the parameters of a common well known illness so that they find themselves in more familiar territory and can offer a treatment with which they have experience. If a medical ward's attending physician becomes convinced that a patient has a particular illness then his error in judgment is passed on to his interns and residents. Then every morning when the physicians and nurses read the patient's chart the first thing they see is the name of the illness that he is asserted to have and this reinforces the general consensus within that ward of that patient's misdiagnosed illness.

A physician must be prepared at all times to challenge the origins of what he considers fact and the minute that anything arises that challenges his knowledge base he must be prepared to dispassionately analyze whether or not the new information should replace the old now outdated information that he currently accepts as the truth. he must routinely question everything and everyone. This unfortunately will not make him very popular.

The most successful physicians usually ignore all previous diagnoses and examine only the primary data in order to develop their own independent diagnosis to compare with any previous ones that may have been offered by other physicians. While others are concentrating on following a well-worn path, the best diagnosis usually comes from the doctor who is able to view the entirety of the peripheral symptoms to arrive at the big picture solution. Which may be quite different from the original diagnosis.

Sometimes the correct diagnosis defies logic and almost becomes intuitive by nature. This type of reasoning is usually based on years and years of experience and the ability to think outside the box. Unfortunately this is an ability that many physicians who have been trained by rote lack or have had beaten out of them by the system. Physicians need to realize that what they think they know can have limitations. They can be blindsided by their training just like any other professional. Physicians can too easily start to rely on their vast knowledge base and overlook the variability factor in human biology.

Adding to these problems is the fact that we understand so little about human biology, which often renders a physician incapable of answering every medical question no matter how qualified he is. An inability to distinguish between personal ignorance or ineptitude and the limitations that are presented by the inadequate advancement of medical science creates another area of uncertainty. All of this uncertainty which is often at a subconscious level can lead to magical thinking on the part of physicians in order to maintain their aura of competence. This characteristic of substituting certainty for uncertainty is not necessarily restricted to doctors but is in general a very human trait. Subconscious falsification of knowledge to protect and enhance one's self-image is more the norm than the exception.

The paradox at the heart of medical decision making is that no matter how meager the data a decision of some sort must be made and acted upon. The training that a physician receives when going through medical school tends to reflect the dogma and knowledge base of the physician who taught him. Those medical students then become doctors who are equally dogmatic in their focus of practicing the antiquated medicine that they learned from that one point of view. Two different medical schools might teach a totally different solution to a particular medical problem, both of which work equally well but none of the medical personnel from those disparate points of view ever get together and discuss which solution might be best for the patient.

Specialization in medicine confers a false sense of certainty. After all the physician is a specialist in that particular area of medical knowledge so he absolutely must project and have confidence in his diagnoses. And once an authoritative senior physician has rendered his decision it becomes an immovable object that impedes the presentation of any other divergent theories that might be more correct. Surgeons vary in their ability to conceptualize the problem and what surgical procedures would or would not be beneficial in that particular instance. The way a surgeon uses his brain is often much more important than how he uses his hands.

The physician must also remember to impart enough information about his diagnosis to the patient so that the patient's expectations for the outcome are not disproportionate to reality. The patient and doctor must be able to communicate sufficiently well that each has a complete understanding of the others expectations about the procedure. There is nothing in biology or medicine that is so complicated that a doctor can not explain it clearly to a patient so that they are able to understand it completely. It has often been said that if you cannot express a concept in words a non-professional can understand then you do not really understand what you're trying to explain. If the physician has an inquiring mind he will continue to improve as he progresses through his career, continually finding innovative techniques to better serve his patients.

Studies have shown that the more error-prone a medical technician is the more certain he is of his diagnosis. The corollary to this is that the dumber a person is the smarter he thinks he is. Radiologists who examine patient x-rays for tuberculosis err 25% of the time. Likewise for breast cancer their error rate is 25% - 40%. Cardiologists misdiagnose EKGs 25% of the time as well. Oncologists who reconsider their own earlier conclusions agree with their first readings only 60% of the time. Senior practitioners only concur with their juniors 50% of the time.

Because of the ever accelerating advances in medical imaging especially in the case of MRIs doctors have a tendency to perform diagnosis by radiologist rather than going through the time-consuming process of developing patient histories. They simply order MRI scans and tell the radiologist to provide them with a diagnosis. It has gotten to the point that physicians expect a definitive answer from the radiologists therefore there is a tremendous pressure on them to come to a very specific conclusion that the doctor can latch onto.

In the United States once a drug has been approved for the treatment of one condition the FDA allows it to be used for the treatment of any other condition if the attending physician so decides. For this reason drug companies have a policy of marketing their drugs directly to physicians by convincing them that it is suitable for the treatment of other more common disorders that have a wider market.

Because of FDA regulations that restrict the drug companies ability to advertise their products for uses other than those that have been specifically approved they tend to use other marketing techniques. Advertisements in popular magazines that are designed to raise awareness of a condition without naming a specific drug is an example. They then try to bully and bribe prominent doctors into using these products for a wider range of treatments as well as urging them to influence other members of their peer group or trainees to use them as well.

While a pharmaceutical company can legally petition the FDA for permission to use a drug to treat other conditions they first need to conducted research trials that indicate efficacy. They seem to get the cart before the horse and do the marketing directly to doctors who are treating that target group of patients. This eliminates the need for expensive research trials to extend the range of uses for the drugs they manufacture.

The opinions of some physicians are faith based rather than science-based. They do not promote various drugs for financial gain but simply because they truly believe in their efficacy. When this belief is backed up by positive clinical studies it is one thing but when it is not it is quite another. There are certain drugs that lend themselves to direct marketing to patients via television and magazines. Usually these are drugs for treating conditions such as arthritis, impotence and erectile dysfunction which are practically impossible to treat to a level at which the patient is satisfied.

Therefore when a new drug is presented to them through advertising they tend to immediately run to their doctor and ask to be prescribed this new drug to see if it will better treat their condition. For such problems as high blood pressure and congestive heart failure there are proven treatments which alleviate most of the symptoms quite effectively and doctors are not as willing to switch from their tried-and-true therapies to something new. This is why you tend to see more advertisements for such things as Viagra and Celebrex rather than for high blood pressure medications.

Quite often physicians who use medical devices and procedures designed and marketed by a particular company receive all expense paid trips to medical conventions being held in exotic locations that are worth thousands of dollars. While physicians who take advantage of these perks claim that they do not influence them to use a particular company's devices or drugs, what may occur is that the number of these procedures increases to the point where many of them may not have been necessary in the first place.

Physicians receive far greater reimbursement for performing a procedure on a patient than they do for the actual physical examination of the patient to determine whether he needs the treatment or not. Overall there is more emphasis on performing invasive surgeries than on using more conservative and equally beneficial procedures. Ruptured vertebrae discs are a good example. Studies indicate that 80% of the patients who decided not to receive vertebrae fusion therapy felt significantly better within six weeks without the surgery. Unfortunately disability insurance payments are much greater when the patient receives back surgery for a work-related injury.

Physicians tend to group maladies that are very complex and resistant to standard therapies under the heading of "difficult to treat." This has a negative psychological affect on physicians by causing them to become resigned to the concept that there's really nothing they can do so they just keep using the same failed procedures that were used in the past rather than sitting down and considering alternative types and directions of attack that might be more beneficial. Doctors tend to be risk-averse and when confronted with these often incurable illnesses are unable to overcome their torpor and take the risk of devising a novel approach. This attitude also acts as a buffer between the physician and his fear of failure. It is this fear of failure that all physicians carry within them that keeps them from attempting new treatments. Unfortunately failure is one of the most prominent aspects of a complicated learning process.

Our knowledge of biology doubles every four years making it almost impossible for physicians to keep up with the major advances in their own area of expertise let alone peripheral fields that directly impact their own. When you add to that the problem of peer pressure to conform to the norm rather than striking out on your own path of discovery you have a formula for substandard patient care. Fear of malpractice suits is another reason that physicians have an aversion to following a path less traveled. Sometimes, however without the risk of failure there is often zero chance of success.

5 HOW OUR IMMUNE SYSTEMS WORK

Malnutrition is the leading cause of immune system deficiency. The proper function of our immune systems can be seriously impaired by the lack of even one vitamin or essential nutrient. Deficiencies of zinc, iron and magnesium for example can result in a serious decreases in T cell numbers and T cell function. This simplified explanation will give you an appreciation of the complexities involved.

There are two parts to our immune systems:

1. **The Passive Immune System:** Which consists of our skin.

2. **The Adaptive Immune System:** Which is the part we will concern ourselves with in this chapter. The adaptive immune system itself has two branches as well, the Humoral and the Cell Mediated. First we will examine the Humoral, which deals with the more liquid areas of our bodies.

The Humoral immune system

Our white blood cells are divided into two main types:

1. **Leukocytes:** Which are nonspecific. This means that they are not programed to locate and kill a specific type of pathogen. When a Leukocyte encounters another cell, it can sense if that cell is in someway defective and kills it.

2. **Lymphocytes:** Which are specific and have been programed to seek out and kill a certain type of pathogen. There are two different types of lymphocytes.

1. **B-Lymphocytes:** They have more than 10,000 protein receptors on the outside of their cell membranes, which are referred to as "membrane bound antibodies". Each B-Lymphocyte has all 10,000 of its' receptors set to the same unique combination of proteins so that there are billions of B-Lymphocytes all with unique protein receptor coding. Our bodies then weed out all of the combinations that would cause the B-Lymphocyte to bond to and kill one of our own normal cells.

When a new type of pathogen enters our body it is continually bumping into the billions of B-Lymphocytes. Eventually it bumps into one whose protein receptors match a protein on the surface of the pathogen causing it to adhere to that B-Lymphocyte's receptor. This triggers a cloning response in that particular B-Lymphocyte and it starts to make copies of itself and since the clones also clone themselves it is not long before there are billions of them.

The odds of a virus bumping into one of these particular B-Lymphocyte clones is now exponentially greater. Now you know why it takes two weeks to get over the flu. First the virus needs to multiply to the point where one of them bumps into the correctly coded B-Lymphocyte. Then that B-Lymphocyte needs time to multiply to the point where there are enough of them to overwhelm the viruses. These billions of newborn B-Lymphocytes then differentiate into two different types:

2. **T-Lymphocytes:** Which are produced in the Thymus. Once again there are two types:

1. **Memory Cells:** Which are passive and just hang out waiting for that same type of pathogen to enter our bodies a second time so that they can kill it immediately instead of going through the whole cloning process all over again. This is why you will never suffer from the same viral infection twice.

2. **Effector Cells:** Which become antibody factories producing 2,000

antibodies per second. These antibodies then attach themselves to any of the associated viruses thereby labeling them for destruction by any Macrophages that happen to encounter them.

The Cell Mediated Immune System

The cell-mediated immune system has two types of cells.

1. **T-Helper Cells:** When they find a part of a pathogen that matches their type of receptor that has been shredded by a B-Lymphocyte or dendritic cell it is mounted to the outside of their cell membrane using a Major Histocompatibility Complex 2 protein base. They then become activated and start cloning themselves into T-Helper memory and T-Helper effector Cells. The T-Helper memory cells function in the same way as the B-Lymphocyte memory cells. The T-Helper effector Cells are slightly different. Instead of producing antibodies they secrete cytokines, which are chemical alarm bells that alert the various parts of our adaptive immune system that they need to start looking for the source of the problem.

2. **T-Cytotoxic Cells:** When a body cell is invaded by a virus or turns cancerous the T-Cytotoxic Cells capture some of the virus's or cancer's protein and displays it on the outside of the infected cell's membrane using an MHC 1 (Major Histocompatibility Complex 1) protein base. This signals that the body cell has that type of pathogen inside of them. When the T-Cytotoxic Cells find a part of a pathogen mounted to the outside of a defective cells membrane they know to kill that cell.

When a T-Cytotoxic Cell finds a body cell displaying an MHC 1 mounted protein that matches its' receptor code it becomes activated and starts cloning itself into T-Cytotoxic memory cells, which like the T-Lymphocyte memory cells live for years in our bodies waiting for the opportunity to attack that same type of pathogen if it ever shows up again. The T-Cytotoxic Cell also clones billions of T-Cytotoxic Effector Cells, which manufacture antigens by the billions as well.

There is a difference between the T-Cytotoxic Effector Cells and the T-Lymphocyte Effector Cells. The T-Lymphocyte Effector Cells inject their antibodies directly into the defective cell instead of releasing them into our bodily fluids to seek out other copies of the pathogen. These T-Cytotoxic Effector Cells are one of our main defenses against cancer.

Inflammatory Response

When our skin is punctured the damaged skin cells signal that they have been damaged by releasing Chemokines to attract our immune system defenses to that location. Mast Cells that are located in the dermal layer of our skin respond to any bacteria or viruses by releasing histamines, which cause our capillaries to dilate in the area where the histamines were released. The dilation causes more separation between the capillary cells so that Neutrophiles and B-Lymphocytes can exit the capillary and attack any bacteria or viruses in the surrounding tissue. Now you know why it is a bad idea to take antihistamines when you have a cold. It prevents this from happening thereby making it more difficult for our immune systems to fight an infection.

Cancer immunotherapy

Neutrophils: Constitute 50-70% of our immune system but can't differentiate between a healthy cell and a cancer cell.

The natural killer cells (NK cells): Are the front line defense against cancer cells but are generic in that they can only detect the difference between a bad cell and a good cell. They do not know why the cell is bad. The question of whether it has been infected by a virus or is cancerous is irrelevant to them. They simply kill any other cell that is diseased for whatever reason. They secrete a substance that eats its way through the cell membrane allowing them to inject granzymes into the cancer cell. These granzymes then reactivate the dormant self-destruct mechanism within the cancer cells. Once dead the cancer cell is consumed by macrophages and eventually eliminated from our bodies.

Cytotoxic T lymphocytes: Unlike the NK Cells these cells are very specialized and are assigned to kill only one type of pathogen and one type only. It might be a virus or a specific type of cancer cell. There are Cytotoxic T lymphocyte helper cells that are also lymphocytes.

They are:

Cytotoxic T 4 lymphocytes: Which are at the top of the command structure and assign tasks to the lower ranked lymphocytes.

Cytotoxic T 8 lymphocytes: Are just below the T4s in the command structure

T helper subset 1 and T Helper subset 2: Are assigned to specific types of pathogens that need killing. These are specific to any virus we have ever had and wait patiently for a recurrence of that virus and the opportunity to kill it.

Cytotoxic T lymphocyte suppressor cells: They keep the other Cytotoxic T lymphocytes from being too aggressive and overloading our other systems by getting the job done too quickly and causing runaway inflammation.

Macrophages: Macrophages are the sanitation workers of our bodies they consume anything that might be harmful by engulfing it. Our white blood cells are the most common type.

A 12 year study of a group of 77 women who already had breast cancer demonstrated the importance of a properly functioning immune system in the elimination of cancer from our bodies. Biopsies of each woman's tumors were cultivated in vitro along with their NK cells. The women were divided into two groups. The first group consisted of patients whose NK cells aggressively attacked their cancer cells. The second group consisted of patients who's NK cells showed little interest in attacking their cancer cells.

From this analysis it appears that the impairment of NK cells in cancer sufferers is approximately 50%. When the study ended 12 years later it was found that half of the patients whose NK cells had failed to attack the cancer cells in the laboratory died of their cancers. 95% of the cancer victims whose immune systems aggressively attacked the cancer cells in the laboratory experiment were still alive after 12 years. This conclusively proves that the old theory that our body's immune system is incapable of attacking cancer cells because they are genetically identical to our normal cells is completely false. Other studies have since verified these results.

Research indicates that cancer routinely fails to establish itself in organisms that have a healthy immune system. The current research studies are starting to focus on strengthening our body's natural defenses against cancer and thereby stabilizing an existing tumor to keep it from enlarging over the long term rather than trying to cut it out or completely destroy it through chemo and radiation. The major actors in this type of therapy are anti-angiogenic medications and nutrients which deny an existing tumor the ability to trick the body into manufacturing blood vessels to feed it.

Inflammation seems to be a major inciting force in both cancer and coronary artery disease. 15% of all cancers can be directly linked to chronic inflammation. Some of the most obvious examples are cervical cancer caused by papilloma virus infection and the Helicobacter pylori bacterium which causes ulcers and stomach cancer. Mesothelioma Is a type of lung cancer caused by inflammation from asbestos exposure. Liver cancer can be caused by the inflammation from hepatitis.

Cancerous growths make use of the inflammatory response by producing the same type of inflammation in the surrounding tissue that would be present if physical trauma had occurred. This tricks the body into thinking that it needs to generate capillaries in that area in order to replace damaged tissue. Instead the capillaries end up feeding the small cancer cell cluster and allowing it to grow into a much larger tumor. Studies have proven that the more successful the cancer is at inducing inflammation in its surrounding area the more aggressively it will be able to expand. Cancer cells are very successful at imitating a normal injury to the body which in turn activates the healing responses such as angiogenesis and the production of cytokines, which cancer cells are very successful at hijacking and utilizing for their own growth and expansion.

Cancer cells essentially produce a wound that never heals. A major factor in this process was recently discovered at the University of California at San Diego. It is called "nuclear factor-kappa B or more commonly NF-kappa B. They have found that blocking this particular factor causes aggressive cancer cells to once again become mortal. Since then it has been determined that nearly every substance that prevents cancer is an inhibitor of the formation of this particular factor. Two of the main sources of these inhibitors are resveratrol and green tea. When the immune system falls into disrepair it stops protecting us from harm. Remember that any good health measure is a good anti-cancer measure as well.

The Immune System and Antibiotics

Your immune System is the only thing that stands between you and the things on you, in you and around you that are trying to kill you. There are only a few types of immune system phages that are capable of recognizing a cancer cell. 80% of your immune system is in your digestive tract and depends on the bacteria there for its effectiveness. Both the antibiotics we take and ones that are residual in dairy and meat products kill those beneficial bacteria. Down here in southern Peru where I currently live I buy my milk fresh and raw from an old lady every morning as I walk back from the gym to my apartment. She has a cow in her back yard, which is located in the middle of the second largest city in Peru! It also is illegal to import GMO produce into Peru. All of the produce is grown and sold locally and is so different in appearance from the US types that it would be obvious if anyone tried to sneak one of the engineered versions into the system here. Never take antibiotics for a viral infection as they are not effective against viruses only bacteria.

Vaccinations and the Immune system

I have never been vaccinated. I am 66 years old and grew up on a subsistence agriculture farm near Springfield, Missouri in the 1950s. Our yearly income was $500 and we didn't even have running water or electricity so vaccinating children was the last thing on anyone's mind. The standard procedure was to expose a child to the main diseases so that he would catch them and develop a natural immunity against it.

Today by 30 months of age a child has had 30 vaccinations some of which contain mercury. Many of these babies are feed commercial formula instead of their mothers' milk so they are not properly nourished and do not receive the immune system boosting benefits of their mother's milk. Children are protected by their mothers immune system until their 6th month and vaccinating them when they are first born is not only futile but detrimental to their health. Their bodies are just too small to deal with it until they are at least one year old.

Dr. Robert Mendelsohn, (1926-1988), who was head of the Pediatric Society and the Chicago Pediatric Hospital, warned against the immunization of babies, many of whom were left with extensive brain damage. Eventually he proved that 85% of Sudden Infant Death Syndrome (SIDS) occurred within 48 hours of a DPT injection, while the remaining 15% of the deaths occurred within 2 weeks of immunization.

6 NUTRITION AND CANCER

Foods and Nutrients that fight Cancer

Unless we are consuming only organically grown food our daily intake of agrochemicals will be extremely high. Many of these chemical contaminants concentrate within our bodies and adversely affect our immune systems abilities to fight off the common cold let alone cancer. Modern food processing only increases the quantity of chemicals contained within the foods we consume. Many of them serve no other purpose than to increase the shelf life and cosmetic appearance of the processed food with no regard to the damage that those preservatives might cause to our bodies. If our immune systems are so impaired that they cannot defeat the common cold than what chance do they have against cancer.

In our quest to acquire sufficient levels of vitamins and nutrients for our bodies we must continually keep in mind that what is offered commercially may not in fact be the correct form of the vitamin that we are seeking to supplement. Vitamin C for instance is not ascorbic acid. The ascorbic acid is only the container for the four or five active ingredients contained in natural vitamin C. It is therefore much more beneficial to receive our vitamin C from natural sources. Likewise vitamin E is usually sold commercially containing only the Alpha portion of natural vitamin E leaving out the beta gamma and Delta portions.

This makes consumption of commercial Alpha vitamin E very detrimental to heart health because the alpha portion when consumed by itself tends to bond with the gamma portions that are already present in our bodies and not allow them to support our hearts. While dying of a heart attack might be the most effective anti-cancer treatment in the short run, for the long run it is probably counter productive.

I included the supplement list from my congestive heart failure book as many of them are anti-carcinogenic as well and will give your heart and immune system much needed support. The statistics are that if cancer does not kill you heart failure will so it is a good idea to be equally proactive in the prevention of both.

Alpha-Lipotic Acid:

The primary function of this nutrient is the restoration of the antioxidant properties of vitamins after they have neutralized free radicals. It is also very beneficial for the liver.

Berries:

Cranberries, Blueberries, Blackberries, Raspberries and Strawberries contain ellagic acid and polyphenols. One of the most effective anti-cancer foods you can eat. Frozen berries are just as potent as fresh.

Broccoli, Brussels Sprouts and Cauliflower: 2 cups per day

These cruciferous vegetables contain Sulfurophane, di-indolylmethane and indole-3-carbinol. Brussels sprouts in particular provide very significant support for the body's detoxification system as well as preventing oxidation and inflammation. Research studies have demonstrated its efficacy against ovarian, prostate, breast and colon cancer. All three of these vegetables contain very high quantities of glucosinolates which are highly protective against the formation of cancer. 2 cups of brussels sprouts provide 500 mg of omega-3 fatty acids about one half of our daily requirement. They are anti-angiogenic and promote cancer cell apoptosis. (Lancet, 2005; 366: 1558–60)

Vitamin C: 1,000mg per day

Double blind studies indicate that 1g per day for 4-6 months significantly reduced blood pressure. It is also a major player in cancer prevention not to mention prevention of scurvy and support of a thousand other metabolic processes.

Conjugated Linoleic Acid (CLA): 1,000mg per day

In one study, mice were fed different amounts of CLA and then were given a carcinogenic chemical that causes breast cancer. 80% of those on a normal diet developed cancer while only 40% given CLA had cancer. A 50% reduction in cancer incidence. Meat and dairy products have always been a good source for this nutrient but modern dairy and livestock practices have so lowered its' levels that supplementation is needed. It promotes body recomposition from fat to muscle. It reduces lipid levels, stops the formation and growth of cancer and stimulates the immune system. This decrease in CLA levels in our foods might be at least a part of the cause of the increases in cancer, heart disease, diabetes, and obesity. This is another reason I moved to South America, the cattle are all free range instead of grain feed and have four times as much CLA in their meat and dairy products.

CoQ10: 300mg per day

Double blind studies indicate that 150mg day decreased BP by 18/12hg after 1-4 months. Also improves cell mitochondrial function. (Southern medical journal 2001;1112-1117)

Citrus fruits: contain flavonoids that detoxify and remove carcinogens from the liver.

Dark chocolate: (Unsweetened with a cacao content of at least 70 per cent) Contains antioxidants and polyphenols that retards the growth of cancer cells (http:// ezinearticles.com/?Dark-Chocolate-Health- Benefits-For-Everyone&id=2422699>).

Vitamin D3: 2,000 iu per day should be enough. Slows the spread of all cancer types by supporting the immune system.

D-Ribose: 5-10g per day

There are no natural sources for this so your body must synthesize it. There is never enough. It is used in our DNA, RNA and ATP. It powers every muscle in our body and is especially important for heart health and function.

Vitamin E: Avocados are the richest source of natural vitamin E.

Do not take the usual form of commercial vitamin E that only contains Alpha-Tocopherol. The other three isomers of natural vitamin E are the Beta, Gama and Delta types of Tocopherol. Gama-Tocopherol is very heart protective but when the Alpha version is ingested by itself it bonds with the Gama-Tocopherol that is already present in our bodies so that there is no free Gama-Tocopherol to help maintain our hearts.

In a recent double blind study of people with risk factors for heart disease who took 400iu of Alpha-Tocopherol vitamin E per day for seven years. There was a 40% increase in the number of hospitalizations and a 19% increase in heart failures over the control group. Not a very good advertisement for taking the Alpha-Tocopherol version of vitamin E! Also be aware that vitamin E and fish oil are also blood thinners, which can cause excessive thinning when used in conjunction with prescription blood thinners. This may allow you to reduce the amount of prescription blood thinner that you need to take. For vitamin E to function properly within our bodies a proper level of zinc must be present as well.

Flax Seeds:

Place 1/4 cup of ground flax seed in a blender with 1-2 cups of yogurt or cottage cheese and blend for one minute. Let it sit for 5 minutes prior to consumption. Flax seed is anti-angiogenic and inhibits the formation of blood vessels by cancer cells to support their growth. Studies have found that flax seeds increase apoptosis in cancer cells by 31%.

Ginger root:

Prevents cancer cell proliferation. Can be consumed as a tea as well as a seasoning. (Cancer Res, 1996; 56: 1023–30).

Green tea: Four cups per day

Contains polyphenols, catechins and epigallocatechin gallate-3, (EGCG). Must be steeped for fifteen minutes to release all of its' polyphenols! Should be consumed within an hour of brewing for full potency.

Herbs and spices:

Especially basil, marjoram, mint, oregano, rosemary and thyme. They block the enzymes that cancer cells need to invade adjacent cells (J Nutr, 2001; 131: 3027S–33S)

L-arginine: 1,000mg per day

Peanuts are 33% arginine by weight. It causes vasodilation, improves cardiac output and Increases endurance and strength. Promotes repair of damaged muscle tissue.

L-carnitine: 1,000mg per day

Improves heart ejection fraction, exercise tolerance and prolongs survival as well as improving fat lose. It also aids in the transport of fatty acids into cells.

Lycopene: 5mg per day.

One of the best reasons to make your own tomato sauce. This antioxidant is primarily found in tomatoes and significantly reduces prostate and colon cancer risk. The tomatoes need to be cooked to release their Lycopene. Also contained in apricots, beets, squash, carrots, and sweet potatoes. (J Natl Cancer Inst, 1999; 91: 317–31;

Magnesium: 500mg per day

Heart Failure patients need about 1,000mg of magnesium per day for the first two months of recovery. CHF patients can only absorb 33% as much serum magnesium into the heart muscle as a healthy person. Use the Gluconate version of Magnesium as it is more readily utilized by the heart. 1-2g of IV magnesium administered weekly for six weeks produced marked improvement in 80% of CHF patients. Most patients maintained the improvement for at least a year. Thousands of bodily functions depend on magnesium.

The proper ratio of calcium to magnesium

The ideal ratio of calcium to magnesium seems to be about 2:1. In order to calculate your correct dosage of supplemental magnesium you will first need to determine your approximate daily intake of calcium. If you do not consume a significant amount of dairy products you can safely supplement 1000 mg of calcium and 500 mg of magnesium. However if you consume a large quantity of dairy products such as cheese and milk you will need to calculate the approximate calcium that you are receiving from them and subtract that from the 1000 mg of calcium supplementation.

The reason for this is that excessive calcium in our systems that is not utilized by biological processes can form kidney stones as well as plaque on the inside of our arteries. Dosages over 500 mg of magnesium on the other hand will usually cause diarrhea in most people. Obviously chronic constipation might be an indication that your intake of magnesium is inadequate. So rather than taking a commercial laxative it would be better to use magnesium instead. You will probably find that you will need to supplement 1,000mg per day for a week to eliminate the constipation and then back off to 500mg per day to prevent it from causing diarrhea. These parameters need to be tailored to the individual so you will have to experiment and come up with a ratio that seems to work best for you.

A proper level of magnesium is vital for the proper utilization of calcium as well as vitamin D by our bodies. Magnesium converts vitamin D into its active form at which point it can assist with the proper absorption of calcium into our bones. Magnesium also stimulates the production of the hormone calcitonin which is utilized by our bodies to draw calcium deposits out of our blood and soft tissues moving them back into our bones where they belong.

This lowers the probability of osteoporosis as well as arthritis, heart attack and the formation of kidney and gallstones. There is growing evidence that systemic inflammation of our vascular system is what actually causes cholesterol and calcium to form plaque on their interiors. So making sure that 100% of the calcium that we consume is properly utilized is essential not only for the health of our bones but our cardiovascular system as well.

Magnesium gluconate is much more readily absorbed by our heart muscle cells which require large quantities of it for proper function so it would probably be best to use that particular type of magnesium. Insufficient magnesium in our diets also contributes to inflammation and oxidation. Potassium is important because it regulates proper heart rhythm, blood pressure, hydration, digestion and muscle cell contraction.

Signs of Magnesium Deficiency

Magnesium is an essential mineral our bodies cannot manufacture so it must be obtained through diet. Most people in the United States have a magnesium deficiency which interferes with nearly 20,000 biological processes within their bodies. What I'm going to provide in this section is some diagnostic tools that you can use to determine if your obtaining sufficient magnesium, calcium and potassium in your diet. Your heart muscle cells contract and relax according to their electrical charge either positive or negative.

In order to create these alternating charges your heart muscle cells must take in and expel magnesium and calcium ions at the same rate that the hearts beats. This requires an incredibly large quantity of these minerals in our blood plasma in order to create the 100,000 pulses per day that our hearts must generate to keep us alive let alone all of the other critical processes that magnesium facilitates throughout our bodies.

Chronic low level stress is one of the main contributors to magnesium deficiency. Whether it is caused by interpersonal relationships, job problems or just the general stress of living in a large city in these modern times, stress is not simply an emotional condition. It also promotes physiological changes within our bodies one of which is the secretion of cortisol. When it becomes impossible for us to resolve the issues which are causing our stress we then have a constant and steady drip of cortisol entering our bloodstream.

This interferes with the proper function of our body by shutting down our immune systems along with countless other biological processes that it considers unnecessary so that we can use that energy for the fight or flight response to danger. 15,000 years ago the stress was over in less than 10 minutes and you were either dead or out of danger. If only it was that simple today. Chronic low level stress is a carcinogen the same as any chemical environmental contaminate.

Another little known cause of magnesium deficiency is diuretics. Drinking several cups of caffeinated coffee each day produces a major loss of magnesium. However on the plus side it also decreases your chance of having cancer by 40% so don't necessarily stop drinking coffee to conserve magnesium just supplement enough magnesium to make up for your magnesium losses and keep the coffee. Obviously if you have congestive heart failure drinking a beverage which causes your blood vessels to constrict might not be a good idea in the first place! In that case substitute green tea.

One possible scenario would be to drink your coffee in the morning then wait a couple of hours until it's out of your system, then take your magnesium supplement and obtain the benefits of it for the remainder of the day. In most of the developed world especially the United States the main contributor to magnesium deficiency is our diets. Mainly because of the high consumption of refined carbohydrates especially sugar as a substitute for proper nutrition.

One of the most prevalent symptoms of magnesium deficiency is depression, which judging by the record sales of antidepressants in the US seems to be at epidemic levels. Another symptom is high blood pressure. Magnesium causes our blood vessels to dilate thereby reducing blood pressure. An insufficiency of magnesium has the opposite effect so if you have high blood pressure one of the first things you do is supplement magnesium and see if that corrects the problem. Another manifestation of low magnesium levels are migraine headaches. In a large percentage of cases supplementation of magnesium eliminates or greatly reduces the frequency of migraines.

If a person has high blood pressure due to low levels of magnesium his cardiologist will assume that it is being caused by his RAA System and will prescribe a diuretic to reduce the quantity of blood that his heart has to pump. The diuretic then reduces the patient's magnesium level even further and produces the opposite of the effect that was intended. Almost everyone knows to supplement calcium as a preventative for bone loss. What they do not realize is that magnesium and calcium are synergistic and must be used together by our bodies to enable many of the benefits that we attribute solely to calcium supplementation. The magnesium is a critical component in the mineralization of the outer hard layers of our bones so you can take all the calcium you want but if you are not at the same time consuming enough magnesium you will still have osteoporosis.

Another indication of low magnesium levels is muscle twitching or spasms. If you have an overly high blood viscosity this can also be caused by low magnesium levels. The easiest way to deal with high blood viscosity levels is to simply donate a pint of blood every three months which will probably be just as effective at thinning your blood as the prescription medications such as warfarin but will be far less detrimental to your health.

Melatonin: 1-3mg prior to sleeping.

Has a very synergistic effect when taken with other anti-carcinogenic nutrients. This one puts you to sleep so it is probably best taken at night prior to bedtime. (Supp Care Cancer, May 1995) (Cancer, 1994; 73: 699–701).

Mushrooms:

Immune System Stimulation. cremini, enokidake, maitake, oyster and portobello. (International Journal of Cancer 15 (2009): 1404-8)

Olive Oil:

Use one tablespoon or more per day for cooking. Extra virgin, cold pressed is the most potent form.

Omega-3 fatty acids: 2g per day.

Ideally our Omega-6 to Omega-3 ratio should not exceed 4:1 (1:1 is perfect). This should not only be achieved through supplementation of Omega-3 but by reduction of Omega-6 as well. Because it is a blood thinner fish oil has modest blood pressure lowering effects.

Onions:

Also chives, garlic, leeks and shallots) promote cancer cell apoptosis. (Cyto technology, 2008; 56: 179–85).

Plums, apricots and Peaches: They provide the same anticancer benefits as Berries. Be sure to eat the kernels as well.

Pomegranate Juice: One cup per day. Anti-inflammatory.

Potassium: 1,000mg per day

High potassium intake lowers BP and protects against hypertensive effects of salt. Suppresses renin release, increases urination, relaxes vascular smooth muscle. Significantly lowers BP. A person's diet contains about 1.5 g. Contraindicated in end stage renal disease and patients taking potassium-sparing diuretics.

PQQ: (pyrroloquinoline quinone) 50 mg daily

Both human and animal studies indicate that PQQ can positively influence both mitochondrial and neural function. In this respect its benefits are very similar to that of resveratrol. It is however 25 to 50 times more potent than resveratrol and is found in a wide variety of foods.

Probiotics:

An occasional dose of probiotics will help your digestive system function at peak efficiency thereby breaking down nutrients more thoroughly and supporting the immune system. Especially important after taking a course of antibiotics.

Resveratrol: 1,000mg per day.

This is the only easily obtainable Supplement that has been proven to lengthen the telomeres on the ends of our DNA thereby lengthening both the quantity and quality of our lives. Recent studies have shown that most of a dose of resveratrol when swallowed is destroyed by the digestive tract.

The proper way to take it is to open the capsule and pour the contents between the lower lip and the lower gum where it will be absorbed directly into your blood stream within about 30 minutes. You can then swallow the rest. This will result in a blood level more than 200 times greater than swallowing the 1,000mg capsule. This is approximately equal to swallowing a half pound of resveratrol.

Selenium: 300 mcg per day

A couple of brazil nuts per day will provide it. It is a critical nutrient for support of the immune system and heart.

Taurine: 1,000mg per day

Actively transported into heart muscle cells at hundreds of times the concentrations found in the blood. This probably means that the heart considers it to be vital for its health. It stabilizes cell membranes and has inotropic and anti-arrhythmic effects. The good news is that four eggs a day will supply enough. Make sure that the eggs are from free range chickens.

Thiamine and B6:

Take a good B complex supplement once a day. Thiamine deficiency can cause congestive heart failure so supplementation is essential. 50mg twice per day is enough. It will increase your body's need for magnesium so be sure to supplement that as well.

Turmeric:

An antioxidant and anti-inflammatory spice which promotes apoptosis in cancer cells. It is also anti-angiogenic. It should be taken with black pepper and olive oil for improved absorption. (Clin Cancer Res, 2008; 14: 4491–9)

Water: 3 liters of purified water per day minimum

Your body needs at least this much per day to function properly on a cellular level. Yes, even water prevents cancer.

Spices that have anti-carcinogenic effects.

Turmeric:

Antioxidant and anti-inflammatory. Reduces excessive cholesterol levels.

Ginger:

Anti-inflammatory and anti-carcinogenic. Aids in the prevention of blood clots.

Garlic:

A source of sulfites which inhibit the growth of tumors. It has also been proven to have antibiotic properties.

Cardamom:

An anti-inflammatory and anti-carcinogen.

Cayenne pepper:

Contains capsaicin which induces cancer cell death by blocking the utilization of proteins required for cancer cell growth and survival.

Chives:

Inhibits the growth of Gastrointestinal cancers.

Nutmeg: Promotes cancer cell apoptosis.

Cilantro: Aids in the removal of heavy metals from our bodies. Extracts of cilantro are routinely used in chelation therapy.

Cinnamon: Protects healthy cells from damage.

Cloves: Protects our skin cells from becoming cancerous.

Black pepper: Anti-angiogenic.

Basil: Studies have shown that basil helps prevent colon cancer.

Parsley: Rich in antioxidants such as vitamin C and beta carotene. Contains Apigenin.

Are you starting to notice a pattern here. All of the above are standard spices that in the past were routinely used for the preparation of foods. Because of the usually bland food that we consume in Western societies today our diets are deficient in the anti-inflammatories and antioxidants that these spices provided in the past and currently provide in Asian cultures. It must however be remembered when supplementing with nutrients and vitamins that too much of a single good thing can be counterproductive. Variety in our daily nutrition is much better for our overall health than fixating on one particular nutrient for which healing properties have been claimed.

Many anticancer nutrients are also synergistic. In other words consumption of several of them together in smaller quantities creates an infinitely greater efficacy than consuming 10 times as much of one of them.

Nutritional Deficiencies That Cause Cancer

Very few people realize how diet influences our susceptibility to both cancer and a multitude of other infirmities. The effects of a poor diet are cumulative and the longer we suffer with poor nutrition the longer it will take to remedy the problems that it has caused. It is infinitely preferable to defeat cancer quickly in its initial stages through proper nutrition than to try and control and eradicate it once it has become detectable and has spread to other areas of our bodies. An ounce of prevention in this case is worth much more than a pound of cure.

We must always be proactive about our health and nutrition. All organisms thrive when they are placed in an environment that is conducive to their growth and cancer cells are no exception. Fortunately the environmental conditions in which cancer cells thrive are substantially different from those of a healthy body. Therefore we must always be certain that the internal chemistry of our bodies is not conducive to the creation and growth of cancer. The first line of defense against any disease is always proper nutrition. After that targeted supplementation of certain nutrients can take our bodies to the next level and make them super resistant to cancer instead of just very resistant.

Another aspect of proper nutrition are the special needs of our brains. The brain is responsible for the consumption of 20% of the oxygen and nutrients that enter our bodies. To function properly neurons require twice as much energy input as any other cell type in our bodies. Brain cells are continually communicating with one another through electrical impulses which cause them to consume large amounts of energy due to their endless signaling. Our brains also manufacture enzymes, hormones and other essential regulatory compounds all of which requires an inordinate amount of energy and nutritional input as well. Proper maintenance of our brains is a primary concern of our bodies so that if we have any deficiencies in nutrients most of those nutrients will be used up in the maintenance of our brain cells leaving a deficit of nutrients for the remainder of our body maintenance.

Omega-6 to Omega-3 Ratio

An interesting clue to the obesity epidemic that is sweeping industrialized countries and the United States in particular, are the changes in Omega-6 to Omega-3 ratios in both dairy and meat products that are being consumed by their populations. Prior to the 1950s dairy cattle were pasture fed and cows gave birth in the spring when those pastures were especially rich in Omega-3 fatty acids which were then concentrated into the cows milk. These Omega-3 fatty acids are also found in the eggs of free range chickens who consume natural foods such as insects.

After the 1950s the demand for both eggs and milk accelerated rapidly with the result that farmers needed to find ways to exponentially increase the productivity of their chickens and cows. Not enough pasture land was available to maintain free range cows and chickens so factory farming was instituted whereby both cows and chickens were fed a diet of corn, soy and wheat. This resulted in eggs and milk that are very high in Omega-6 fatty acids. The end result is that our diets now contain an excess of Omega-6 fatty acids and almost no Omega-3. The imbalance is quite often more than 30:1 in favor of the Omega-6.

The correct ratio for proper health is 1:1. Omega-6 fatty acids stimulate the production of fat cells from the moment of our birth until we die. Omega-3 helps with the development of our nervous systems and increase the pliability of cell membranes while reducing inflammation and limiting the production of fat cells.

Cows are also injected with estradiol to keep them producing milk for a longer period of time with the result that the estradiol ends up in the milk itself and when fed to babies and infants causes them to produce a greater quantity of fat cells. Other hormones that are routinely injected into cows to increase their milk production cause an increase in systemic Insulin-like Growth Factor, which is then concentrated into the milk and is not destroyed by pasteurization. This results in the increased stimulation of fat cell production as well as inflammation. This is why only their mothers natural milk should be used to nurse babies.

During the 1960s the US government started promoting the use of margarine instead of butter. The problem is that the hydrogenated trans-fats that are used to produce margarine are rich in omega six fatty acids some of which contain more than 50 times as much Omega-6 as Omega-3. This makes it almost impossible to achieve the preferred one to one ratio of Omega-3 to Omega-6 even through Omega-3 supplementation. This has produced a worldwide epidemic of systemic inflammation which contributes to the increase of cancer and cardiovascular disease. Israel because of its dietary laws has one of the lowest cholesterol levels of all western countries but with the highest rate of myocardial infarction and obesity.

Practical Food Quality Solutions

Livestock that are raised under modern factory feed lot conditions and fed high corn, wheat and soy diets produce meat , that is very low in Omega-3 fatty acids. However when as little as 5% flaxseed is introduced into their diets the quality of the food products derived from them increases exponentially. In a study designed to test the efficacy of this approach one group of animals was fed the normal diet of corn, wheat and soy. The second group received the same diet but with the addition of 5% flaxseed. Two groups of people were then formed. One group consumed only the food products from the group of animals whose diet included the flaxseed. The other group of people consumed only the food products from the other group of animals whose diet did not include the flaxseed.

After three months all of the people who participated had their blood tested to determine their ratios of Omega-3 to Omega-6 fatty acids. The participants who ate the food products from animals who consumed flaxseed had three times the level of omega-3 fatty acids as did the other group who consumed food products from the animals who had not been fed flaxseed.

Two years later the researchers repeated their study using obese diabetics. The group of diabetics who consumed the food products derived from animals who's diets had included flax had an average weight loss of 3 pounds even though they had consumed exactly the same number of calories as the control group. The researchers also hired an independent laboratory to conduct taste testing of the two different types of animal products the majority of participants selected the omega-3 rich foods as being better tasting than the ones that were poor in omega-3 content. (http://www.bleu-blanc-coeur.org/files/2002_Annals_Nutrition_Metabolism _Effects_of_introducing_Weill.pdf)

7 CARCINOGENS

Aspartame

A recent research study shows that aspartame use causes an increased risk of leukemia and myeloma. Another 22 year study by Dr. Eva Schernhammer demonstrated that the consumption of one or more carbonated beverages per day containing aspartame caused a serious increase in blood cancers. Another research study published in the American Journal of Clinical Nutrition has indicated the same connection between carbonated aspartame sweetened beverages and blood cancer.

Carcinogenic fats

Western diets are so rich in Omega-6 fatty acid foods that it is almost impossible to achieve the preferred 1 to 1 ratio of Omega-6 to Omega-3 even through the use of Omega-3 supplements. This has produced a Western epidemic of systemic inflammation which contributes to the increase of cancer and cardiovascular disease.

The margarine-based source of hydrogenated vegetable oils (HVOs) is fairly easy to avoid. All we need to do is use butter instead of margarine. The real problem here is the pervasive use of HVOs in processed foods such as pastries, potato chips, cookies and crackers. The hydrogenation process makes these vegetable oils less digestible and more inflammatory than those oils that occur naturally.

HVO's have one big advantage for the manufacturer of processed foods. They never become stale therefore the products made from them have a very long shelf life. The annual consumption of HVO's has increased from 1 pound in 1935 to more than 24 pounds in 2015. The prevalence of both cancer and coronary disease as well as obesity have increased at about the same rate over the same period of time.

A recent study conducted by the French national Institute for health showed that women who consume high amounts of HVO's have twice as many cases of breast cancer as women who consume low amounts of trans-fats. A very large research study in the late 90s demonstrated that the polyunsaturated fats used to make margarines and vegetable oils significantly increase the risk of cancer. These test results also showed that the use of monounsaturated fats such as olive oil decreases the risk of cancer. Likewise the consumption of saturated fat was found not to be a risk factor for cancer.

Overall our consumption of polyunsaturated fats has tripled over the last century while the consumption of other types of fat has remained about the same. The reason for this is that we were told that it is healthier. In reality our bodies are made up of only 3% polyunsaturated fat the majority being monounsaturated at 55% and saturated at 42%. Unfortunately most people's diets provide them with a fat intake, which is 30% polyunsaturated oils. The reality is that we only require a 5% caloric intake of polyunsaturated fats.

One problem with high consumption of polyunsaturated fats is that our bodies can use them for purposes they are not appropriate for such as the construction and repair of cell membranes for which saturated fats are normally used. Because polyunsaturated fats are very unstable and easily damaged by the sun's ultraviolet light free radicals can be formed which damage the cells DNA causing skin cells to become cancerous. Hydrogenated fats are another type of fat that we should avoid. They result in inflammation and the formation of free radicals at the cellular level. This type of fat is usually found in commercial baked goods such as: cookies, cakes, margarine, fried food, crackers and snack foods.

Once considered unsafe to eat, saturated fats have recently been reinstated as the healthy choice for their abilities to remain stable and not form free radicals. The best of the saturated fats are the medium chain triglycerides such as those found in coconut oil and avocados. The consumption of coconut oil increases the effectiveness of our immune system's TNF hormone (Tumor Necrosis Factor) by 60 times. Coconut oil also contains palmitic acid, which is a very effective anticancer agent. Many of the countries that have very low cancer rates use coconut oil for cooking. Recent studies have shown that most of the arterial clogging is caused not by saturated fats but by unsaturated and polyunsaturated fats.

Trans-fats

Trans-fats are created by heating vegetable oil to a very high temperature at which point it becomes solid rather than liquid. The advantage for processed food manufacturers is that it has a very long shelf life and can easily be incorporated into processed foods in a manner that speeds production. This is great for the manufacturers bottom line but unfortunately not so good for the consumer who has to eat a product which is essentially toxic to our bodies causing systemic inflammation heart problems and obesity as well as having been proven to increase infertility in women.

But the main problem with the consumption of trans-fats is that our bodies normally use saturated fat for cell membrane repair and creation. If there are insufficient quantities of saturated fat for our bodies to use for cell membrane maintenance they will use trans fats and polyunsaturated fats instead. This creates membranes that are very inflexible and not as permeable to osmosis as when they are made from saturated fats.

Cellphones

Cellphone use is pervasive throughout modern society. Nearly everyone has one and uses it daily if not hourly. The electromagnetic field generated by the cell phone when it is being used as well as the cell phone tower emissions quite often need to pass through your head and brain depending upon the physical relationship between the cell phone tower and your cell phone. Young people are especially susceptible since they tend to spend hours per week communicating by cell phone with their friends.

One of the problems with obtaining reliable data about cell phone caused cancer is that many of the studies that have exonerated cell phone usage as a cause of cancer were paid for by the cell phone manufacturing industry. It is not difficult to imagine that if micro seconds of accumulated x-ray exposure can cause cancer in healthy individuals then perhaps hours of exposure to radiation that is of a slightly lower frequency can also have adverse effects on our brains. Here's a list of independent research studies which seem to verify that cell phone usage does cause brain tumors.

The greater the usage of cell phone the greater the risk of developing cancer.(Int J Occup Saf Ergon, 2007; 13: 63–71)

The younger the user the greater the risk. (Arch Environ Health, 2004; 59: 132–7).

The risk of brain cancer is increased by 5% for every hundred hours of cell phone usage. (Int J Occup Saf Ergon, 2007; 13: 63–71).

Yearly usage of a cell phone is cumulative and seems to increase the risk of brain tumors by 8% per year of usage. (Int J Occup Saf Ergon, 2007; 13: 63–71).

Persons who have used a cell phone for more than 10 years have nearly a 300% greater chance of brain tumors over people who have used a cell phone for fewer years.(Int Arch Occup Environ Health, 2006; 79: 630–9).

The greater the level of radiation produced by the cell phone the greater the risk. (Occup Environ Med, 2005; 62: 390–4).

There is a three times greater risk of cerebral tumors occurring on the same side of the head as a cell phone is used on. The odds of that malignancy occurring in young people who start using a cell phone before the age of 20 is five times greater. (Int J Oncol, 2009; 35: 5–17)

Many research studies have indicated a much greater danger for young users of cell phones than for adults. This seems logical sense their physiology is still developing. A good source for further information is www.radiationresearch.org they Also have an excellent guide with tips on how to minimize the effects of cell phone radiation on your health. There are a number of things you can do to limit your exposure to microwave radiation from cell phones.

When you have a weak signal from the tower avoid using your phone because it will go into high-power mode and expose you to a stronger signal. Obviously using the text messaging feature rather than voice will expose you to an exponentially smaller amount of radiation as well as duration. You should also regularly switch ears when speaking to someone to limit the amount of exposure in one area of your brain.

Chemical Carcinogens

If you do not believe that fluoride is a poison then you should read the warning label on the back of your toothpaste tube. Although it is somewhat beneficial for preventing tooth decay if applied topically to teeth it is a very serious poison if swallowed. Contained within the fluoride are small amounts of mercury, lead, beryllium and arsenic. Dr. Dean Burke who was employed as a chemist by the National Cancer Institute stated that "fluoride causes more cancer deaths, faster than any other chemical."

Some of the side effects of fluoride intake include osteoporosis, birth defects and kidney ailments. Research studies have indicated that as the use of fluoride increases so does oral and bone cancer. According to the handbook of toxicology of commercial products fluoride is considered to be more poisonous than lead. Like lead fluoride is cumulative and readily absorbed by our bones. Fluoride is considered an environmental toxin if it accidentally finds its' way into rivers or lakes. Why then is it considered to be beneficial if deliberately added to our drinking water.

Research studies have proven time and again that the consumption of red meat itself does not cause cancer. It is only when sodium nitrate and potassium nitrite are added to it that it becomes carcinogenic. Organic foods are never used by the health and food industries when they perform their own research studies because they will provide the wrong results for what those industries are trying to prove. Commercially grown chickens are always fatter than free range ones because they never get any exercise and they are fed arsenic as a fattening agent. This was approved by the FDA in 1944.

Artificial fertilizers are no substitute for crop rotation. This is even more effective when animals are grazed on the same land and their droppings then plowed into the soil to increase its' fertility. This has been standard procedure for thousands of years before the production of chemical fertilizers which were first introduced 150 years ago. Many of the chemicals currently used not only reduce the fertility of the soil and contaminate it with carcinogens but also kill the microorganisms, which are so beneficial for breaking down the organic material in soils.

Plants raised in soil that has been depleted of its nutrients are so weakened that they are incapable of protecting themselves from insect and fungal attacks. Likewise the bodies of humans who subsist on those plants then lack the nutrients needed to prevent cancer from forming. Unfortunately after a couple of years of use the insect population develops an immunity to that particular insecticide and newer more lethal ones need to be introduced to handle the problem. Unfortunately humans are unable to develop this resistance and suffer disproportionately as a result. This is especially true of children whose immune systems have not yet fully developed and have less body mass to absorb the toxins.

The pesticides DDT and DDE interfere with male production of testosterone thereby greatly reducing fertility in any population where it's used. These pesticides are always concentrated in the breast tissue of mothers who are feeding their infant's. This results in a higher rate of breast cancer as well as a higher cancer rate among infants and young children.

Eventually all of these agricultural chemicals find their way into rivers which then flow into the oceans. Most of them do not decompose and are bio-accumulative. They are concentrated in plankton and other small organisms. When these plankton are consumed by crustaceans and other larger organisms they concentrate that poison within themselves. The crustaceans such as shrimp are then consumed by even larger predator fish who are then contaminated to an even higher level. When these smaller fish are then consumed by very large predator animals such as seals and large game fish the concentration of poisons within them is exponentially higher.

Despite their pristine arctic environment the polar bears have one of the highest chemical contamination levels of any mammal on earth simply because their food source is large fish and seals who themselves are contaminated by their own food source. The consumption of large game fish such as tuna and swordfish is probably not a good idea because of this and especially now due to the radioactive contamination that is being leaked into the oceans by Fukushima and the vast petroleum contamination of the gulf region by oil spill about five years ago. Most of these chemicals are fat soluble and tend to be concentrated in the fat of the fish and mammals that consume them.

When we consume those fish their chemical contaminants are transferred to our fat stores. These are referred to as persistent organic pollutants by the researchers who study them. Recently an entirely new area of cancer research referred to as environmental oncology was born. It has been found that chemicals when introduced into the body have a compounding effect. In other words although there may be relatively small amounts of each chemical contaminant their effects are synergistic and do more real harm to our bodies than what would be assumed by the small quantities of each individual poison. What is considered an acceptable dose of a single pesticide might cause no problem but the effect of a very minimal dose of 10 Pesticides can prove fatal.

During World War II manufacturing technology was forced to grow at a greatly accelerated pace in order to produce more efficient weapon systems. One facet of this was an increased interest in the production of plastics from petroleum products. Since 1930 the production of synthetic chemicals for industry has grown from 1,000,000 tons per year to more than 200 million tons today. Many of these chemicals when released into the environment do not decay or degrade and become persistent contaminants within every plant and animal living in that environment.

At this point we have probably reached peak contamination of our environment. Because of the ongoing education of the population in general particularly through the Internet people are waking up to the problem and are starting to become more proactive in the fight against all forms of pollution both environmental and biological. Hopefully this will continue and result in a final solution to cancer and heart disease that is biological rather than chemical in nature. Chemical pesticides are not necessary. The runoff from them contaminates fruits, vegetables and other crops not to mention the water supply

Diabetes and Cancer

It has not been until recently that oncologists have begun to understand that high levels of insulin are carcinogenic. Previously they had thought that obesity itself was a cause of cancer. Although fat in and of itself is highly inflammatory to our bodies because of the very high metabolic rate at which it is stored in fat cells and when it is utilized for energy.

Hyperinsulinaemia (over production of insulin) can lead to obesity because insulin converts all of the glucose in our blood to fat. Insulin has a secondary function as well, it stimulates cellular growth by producing insulin-like growth factor (IGF). This process allows our bodies to produce more muscle mass when stimulated by exercise. Unfortunately this stimulation also causes abnormally rapid growth of cancer cells. Cancer cells also have 10 times as many insulin receptors as do normal cells. (Neoplasia, 2009; 11: 672–82) (Cell Commun Signal, 2009; 7: 14)

Instead of obesity being the cause of cancer, both the cancer and the obesity are caused by an excess of insulin production. There is ample proof that type II diabetes caused by insulin resistance and overproduction can be cured in a matter of weeks by simple changes in the foods that we consume. By simply eliminating high glycemic carbohydrates from our diets our insulin production will return to normal levels and as a side benefit very rapid fat loss will occur at the same time. The over consumption of high glycemic foods creates two problems, obesity and high insulin levels leading to cancer cell proliferation.

A study conducted by Harvard medical school on a group of

500 women demonstrated that the ones who consumed the most carbohydrates were three times more likely to develop breast cancer compared to the women who consumed the lowest amounts. (Cancer Epidemiol Biomarkers Prev, 2004; 13: 1283–9)

Another research study indicated that women with higher levels of insulin were more likely to develop breast cancer than women with lower levels. (J Natl Cancer Inst, 2009; 101: 48–60).

There are a total of 40,000 new cases of cancer per year in the United States which may be related to obesity. (Cancer Detect Prev, 2003; 27: 415–21)

Since more than 33% of adults in the US are now classified as obese this connection between deaths from obesity and deaths from cancer caused by high insulin levels are a major health problem. Quantitatively the amount of obesity in the United States is increasing by 1% per year.

The main difference between a person who is lean and one who is obese is that the lean person secretes the correct amount of insulin to optimize his blood glucose level whereas an obese person secretes much more insulin which then moves the blood glucose into the fat cells through a process called lipogenesis rather than burning it to produce energy. Only a very small reduction in carbohydrate intake is needed to produce a significant drop in blood insulin levels.

Estrogen Replacement Therapy

Estrogen is carcinogenic. One of its purposes is to increase the rate of cell division during pregnancy when the levels of estrogen increase dramatically. This has recently become apparent in studies of older women who are on estrogen replacement therapy. Studies have determined that after five years of ERT the likelihood of lung cancer increases by 60%. Obviously the women who are most vulnerable are ones who smoke as well as being on estrogen replacement medications. They also increase their risk of ovarian cancer by nearly 40%. (JAMA, 2009; 302: 298–305)

Food Additives

The chemistry used to produce food additives is so highly developed at this point that any taste or aroma can be artificially produced. Unfortunately these artificial flavors and smells are there to hide the fact that the basic ingredients used to produce that food have no nutritional value at all.

Most of these additives are strictly cosmetic in nature and are used to promote the sale of the product, its shelf life and its profitability. The most commonly used food additives are sodium nitrate, artificial sweeteners, artificial colors and flavors, emulsifiers, thickening agents, monosodium glutamate and very high levels of salt or sugar.

Our bodies react to these poisons by becoming fatigued. They also produce emotional issues such as mood swings and can even lead to heart disease and cancer. The artificial sweetener aspartame is especially attractive to people who enjoy sweets because it has 0 calories. They would probably be less enthusiastic about consuming it if they knew that its first use was as an ant poison.

The FDA which normally rubber stamps any request for approval from the food industry refused to approve aspartame for eight years because they considered it unsafe for human consumption. It only became licensed for use in foods in the early 1980s over the objections of many well known biologists.

Aspartame contains phenylalanine which can produce serious neurological problems. And judging by the epidemic of obesity it doesn't even accomplish its stated goal of helping people control their weight. Many people who seem to suffer from depression and have pre-diabetic conditions as well as arthritis and panic attacks are cured of their symptoms after eliminating aspartame from their diets.

Monosodium glutamate

Monosodium glutamate is a flavor enhancer that was developed at the turn of the 19th century by a Japanese food chemist. Since then it has found its way into nearly every type of processed food. It is highly addictive, increasing a person's consumption of whatever foods contain it thereby increasing the manufacturer's sales. The injection of monosodium glutamate into research rats triples the production of insulin by their pancreases. Some people are so allergic to MSG that it produces a life-threatening reaction in them.

Never consume any commercial artificial sweetener. Although they may reduce your consumption of calories they will not reduce the amount of fat on your body. The only sweetener that I use is stevia. You will be amazed at how sweet vegetables taste once you have abstained from the consumption sugar for a couple of weeks. Once you have overcome your addiction to sugar you will discover why people at the turn of the 19th century only consumed 5 pounds of it per year. It is just not necessary to sweeten your food which is naturally sweet enough without the addition of sucrose.

There is much debate about whether or not the consumption of meat products causes cancer. If the animal that was the source of the meat was raised organically without the use of hormone injections to increase productivity the meat products will not be carcinogenic if only moderate amounts are consumed. This assumes that sodium nitrite was not used as a preservative. While many research studies have shown that Asian cultures who consume very low quantities of meat and Large quantities of vegetables have exponentially lower cancer rates than Western societies we cannot necessarily draw a direct correlation that meat itself produces cancer. Cancer research studies recommend an ideal weekly goal of about 10 ounces or less of red meat in our diets. Even this low limit allows for at least three steak dinners per week.

A better goal would seem to be moderation in everything and excess in nothing. The one absolute concerning our selection of meat products is that they must always come from pasture fed animals. This will assure that the meat we consume has a high level of Omega-3 fatty acids. Since the corn and soy normally used to fatten cattle quickly is associated with very high use of fertilizers, insecticides and herbicides.

One of the things to keep in mind when selecting organic foods at the market is that the term organic only means that the animal was fed grains that were organic. If those animals were not free range and consumed grass as a major part of their food source then they will not produce food products which are healthy. This is why eggs have such a bad reputation for cholesterol. The eggs that were used in the research studies 40 years ago which showed that they contained too much bad cholesterol used powdered eggs from chickens who were raised in cages and fed grains.

Genetically Modified Organisms

Genetically Modified Organisms are Plants or animals that have had genes from another species spliced into them. There are currently six main crops that are being modified. These include field corn, soybeans, cotton, canola, sugar beets, and alfalfa. The two main modification categories are:

1. **Herbicide Tolerant Crops:** Plants with this genetic modification are highly resistant to Roundup Herbicide, This makes weeding easier for farmers because they can simply spray the crops along with the

weeds with no worry of killing the crops.

2. **Endogenous pesticide Producers:** Monsanto takes a bacterium from the soil called Bacillus Thuringiensis and splices its genetic material into the plant they want to protect from insects. When insects consume the plant the toxin produced by the bacteria's genetic material causes perforations in their intestinal and stomach walls and causing them to die.

There are three basic types of seeds heirloom, hybridized and genetically modified. We first need to understand the difference between these three varieties. Seed companies have always had a serious problem with their business paradigm. A farmer only needed to purchase the seeds for a particular crop once. He would then save enough seeds from each crop he grew to grow the next one.

This worked very well for the farmers but not so well for the seed companies. Using this paradigm the seed companies could only sell a particular seed to a particular farmer once, afterwards he ceased to be a customer for that seed. The seed companies could not patent a heirloom seed because it is a part of nature so they were not creating something new and original for which a patent could be issued.

The workaround that the seed companies developed was to set up research departments within their companies to produce hybrid varieties of the various cash crops that had characteristics which would favorably distinguish their products in the marketplace. Their sweet corn might be sweeter than their competitors or their hybrid tomatoes a different color or more flavorful. This worked out for everyone as it created a much greater variety of produce that could be tailored to different tastes and uses.

Every time a seed company developed a new hybrid that was better than the previous one the farmers had to repurchase their seeds to remain competitive in the marketplace. This was a very fair system that benefited everyone from the seed producer to the end customer who had a more flavorful product to put in his salad. But the seed companies still could not patent those hybrid seeds because even though they were different the difference had been derived from the combination of two naturally occurring plants through cross-pollination which occurs naturally as well as in the laboratory.

In 1999 Monsanto hired the Arthur Anderson Consulting Group to help them set up a business plan. The Monsanto executives told the consultants that within 20 years they wanted to genetically modify and patent 100% of all commercial seeds and at the same time eliminate all of the naturally occurring ones. By working backwards from that goal and using that time period of about 20 years the consulting company presented a plan to Monsanto that would provide them with 100% control of all commercial seeds and provided for the virtual extinction of all naturally occurring commercial seed types.

A very necessary ingredient in this whole process was Monsanto's influence within the US and UK governments. This allowed them to monetarily encourage strategic politicians within the various governments to promote Monsanto's plan with sufficient speed that it would not allow grassroots resistance to grow quickly enough to obstruct their program. They wanted the produce markets to become so saturated with genetically modified produce that there would literally be nothing that the consumers could do to eliminate it.

The genetic modification of produce is not so much a conspiracy as it is a logical extension of what is considered good business practice in this modern age. The fact that the total destruction of plant biodiversity should be considered a viable business plan is far more terrifying for me than any conspiracy theory. Monsanto now owns 25% of all of the worlds seed companies and is in the process of buying the remainder. Unfortunately for the biotech companies consumer resistance occurred sooner and was exponentially greater than what they assumed it would be.

So what are the effects on humans who consume Bacillus Thuringiensis and Roundup resistant plants? Monsanto promised that Bacillus Thuringiensis was safe because it only affected certain insects. That turned out to be a lie. The BT toxin in its natural form, which was used as a spray in organic agriculture as well, has been linked to inflammation, compromised immune systems and also tissue damage in mice. More recent studies have found that BT toxin causes perforations in human cells and has been linked to cancer as well as autism, autoimmune disease, food allergies, inflammation in general, Alzheimer's and Parkinson's disease.

The FDA does not require any safety trials of GMOs. In 1992 the white House launched an inquiry into the safety of GMOs. The former attorney for Monsanto, Michael Taylor, oversaw it. The FDA gave him a special position that was designed for him when the agency was told by the White House to promote GMOs. The policy report that he created falsely claimed that the FDA wasn't aware of any information indicating that GMO crops were significantly different from any others therefore no testing or labeling was necessary. Michael Taylor then became Monsanto's vice president and chief lobbyist and later returned to the FDA as the US food safety czar. This has to be the ultimate fox guarding the henhouse scenario.

Companies like Monsanto can now unilaterally conduct their own safety trials, the actual results of which are kept secret, and they of course inform us that GMOs are completely safe. The problem is that Monsanto also told us agent orange, PCBs and DDT were safe as well. A law suit that forced 44,000 secret FDA memos into the public domain showed that the overwhelming consensus among the scientists working at the FDA was exactly the opposite of what the FDA and Monsanto had claimed. The scientists had insisted that GMOs needed to be studied more thoroughly and urged their superiors to require testing. Their concerns were studiously ignored.

The safety tests that Monsanto conducted on animals ended after 90 days and they declared GMO foods to be safe for human consumption. An independent research team decided to extend the 90 day study for two years, the approximate lifespan of the rats being used in the trials. At four months the rats started to grow tumors and by the and of the two years 80% of the female rats had mammary gland tumors and 50% of the male rats developed tumors as well compared to far lower numbers in the control group. It is obvious that Monsanto used pretesting to determine when the rats would start to develop tumors and then terminated the public tests a month earlier to prevent that knowledge from becoming public.

GMOs do cause genetic damage to DNA, which can result in cancer. There are several ways that Roundup promotes cancer. First of all it acts as an antibiotic, which kills beneficial intestinal bacteria allowing an overgrowth of detrimental bacteria. These bad bacteria have been linked by research studies to the propagation of colorectal cancer. Roundup also damages a set of enzymes called the CYP enzymes, which are part of our bodies' detoxification process. When damaged these CYP enzymes promote cancer growth. Roundup is now being used as a ripening agent for all sorts of grains, beans, fruits and vegetables. It's used for sugarcane, barley, rye, lentils, potatoes, sweet potatoes, berries and citrus groves. About the only sure way to avoid glyphosate is to go organic and hope for the best.

In another interesting Canadian study they found the BT toxin in the blood of 93% of pregnant women as well as 80% of their unborn fetuses. Since BT Toxin metabolizes quickly the researchers concluded that the women must have had frequent exposure to it although they were unable to determine the source. A more viable and frightening explanation is provided by the only GMO research study to be conducted on humans.

These Canadian researchers fed their subjects soybeans that contained the Bacillus Thuringiensis genetic modification and found that the BT toxin gene that was inserted into the soybeans was transferring itself into the DNA of bacteria living inside the test subjects' intestines. It has not been conclusively proven but is very possible that once the gene transfers to those bacteria it might cause them to produce the BT toxins which may result in these toxic proteins being produced continuously in our digestive tracts. As soon as the pro-GMO UK government who was funding the study found out about this development the funding was stopped. Perhaps the pregnant women tested in Canada had it in their blood because they are producing it internally within their own digestive systems.

On October 31, 2005 at a conference of the American Academy of Environmental Medicine (AAEM) held in Tucson, AZ. the results of a Russian rat study were presented which showed that 55% of the offspring of female rats fed genetically engineered soy flour died within three weeks. The female rats had received 5-7 grams per day of the Roundup Ready variety of soybeans, beginning two weeks before conception and continuing through nursing. By comparison, only 9% of the offspring of rats fed non-GM soy died. Furthermore, offspring from the GMO-fed group were significantly stunted 36% weighing less than twenty grams after two weeks, compared to only 6% from the non-GMO soy control group.

The board of the American Academy of Environmental Medicine reviewed the Russian research, and endorsed a resolution at their October 30 meeting, which states: "We recognize that this study is preliminary in nature. It hasn't yet been peer reviewed and the methodology has not been spelled out in detail. But given the magnitude of the findings and the implications for human health, we urge the National Institutes of Health to immediately replicate the research." According to Dr. Jim Willoughby, the Academy president, "Genetically modified soy, corn, canola, and cottonseed oil are being consumed daily by a significant proportion of our population. We need rigorous, independent and long-term studies to evaluate if these foods put the population at risk."

The Institute for Responsible Technology in Iowa, presented the AAEM conference with results from other published studies as well. Animals fed GM food developed potentially precancerous cell growth, stunted organs as well as damaged immune systems. According to these studies, the process of gene insertion can turn genes off, permanently turn others on, change the expression of hundreds of other genes, create mutations, and introduce new allergenic proteins.

High Glycemic Index Foods and Cancer

High glycemic index ingredients are mainly found in processed food products. These include all forms of sweeteners especially sucrose (white sugar) as well as white rice and white flour. Because foods with high glycemic index values are turned into glucose much more rapidly than low glycemic index foods such as green vegetables they tend to increase our blood sugar levels and cause the release of large quantities of insulin. Both of these conditions are extremely inflammatory. In 1890 the average person in America consumed less than 5 pounds of sugar per year. Our current yearly consumption is more than 100 pounds per person.

A very important factor in determining a food's glycemic index is the amount of processing that was used in its' production. Using grains as an example milling removes the fibrous outer bran and the vitamin and mineral rich germ leaving common white flour with only the starchy endosperm. If you must consume flour make certain that It was made from whole grains and contains all of the constituents that the original whole grains contained.

All high Glycemic Index Foods cause our blood sugar to spike. Since all cancer cells are "obligate glucose feeders" and can derive their energy from no other source it is probably not a good idea to follow a dietary regime that perpetually elevates blood glucose levels. The high level of blood glucose forces the pancreas to release equally large quantities of insulin along with insulin like growth factor which stimulates rapid cell growth. Both glucose and insulin are two of the worst inflammatory agents in our bodies and greatly contribute to the systemic inflammation that causes both cancer and heart disease.

In one study two groups of mice were inoculated with breast cancer cells and divided into two groups one of which was fed a high glycemic diet and the other a very low glycemic diet. After 75 days two thirds of the high glycemic diet mice died from cancer. In the other low glycemic group only one mouse out of the 24 died from the cancer.

A study that compared Asian and Western populations found that those who consume low sugar Asian and Mediterranean diets have seven times fewer cancers which are caused by hormonal issues then people in industrialized countries who subsist on a diet high in sugars. Likewise many other studies have conclusively drawn the same connection between the consumption of high glycemic foods and the prevalence of prostate and breast cancer as well as colon and ovarian cancer.

Obesity and Cancer

Obesity may be the direct cause of may illnesses and might contribute to the growth of cancer as well through the overproduction of the hormone Aromatase. Many hormones are produced by our adipose tissue, the quantity produced being dependent upon our percentage of body fat. One of these hormones is Aromatase, whose function is to convert testosterone into estrogen. This is one of the reasons that women need to have a minimum of 15% body fat to maintain hormonal balance.

Likewise excessive fat creates an excess of estrogen in men, which causes ever more production of fat and damage to their hormonal balance. Estrogen also promotes cell proliferation in existing cancers as well. Estrogen is a carcinogen in that its presence greatly accelerates cell division. This is why during pregnancy women produce more estrogen than normal. This higher level of estrogen is needed to increase the rate of cell division within the fetus.

A major cause of the current obesity epidemic especially in the United States is the use of high fructose corn syrup as a sweetener. A study conducted by George Brey and his colleagues at the Louisiana State University found that HFCS consumption leads to leptin resistance. Leptin is a hormone that tells our brain that we have eaten enough and our stomach is full. When it is inhibited we tend to eat more because we continually feel hungry.

As has been previously stated prior to the 1950s dairy cattle were pasture fed and cows gave birth in the spring when those pastures were especially rich in omega-3 fatty acids which are then concentrated into the cows milk. These omega-3 fatty acids are also found in the eggs of free range chickens who consume natural foods such as insects. After the 1950s the demand for both eggs and milk accelerated rapidly with the result that farmers needed to find ways to exponentially increase the productivity of their chickens and cows.

Not enough pasture land was available to maintain free range cows and chickens so factory farming was instituted whereby both cows and chickens were fed a diet of corn, soy and wheat. This resulted in eggs and milk that are very high in omega six fatty acids. The end result is that our diets now contain an excess of omega six fatty acids and almost no omega-3's. The imbalance can be as high as

30:1 in favor of Omega six. The ideal ratio for good health is 1:1. Omega six fatty acids stimulate the production of fat cells from the moment of our birth until we die. The omega threes help with the development of our nervous systems, increase the pliability of cell membranes, reduce inflammation and limit the production of fat cells.

Cows are also injected with estradiol to keep them producing milk for a longer period of time with the result that the estradiol ends up in the milk itself and when fed to babies and infants causes them to produce a greater quantity of fat cells. Other hormones that are routinely injected into cows to increase their milk production cause an increase in systemic IGF which then passes into the milk and is not destroyed by pasteurization. This results in the increased stimulation of fat cell production as well.

Oncologists have long thought, and many of them still do, that obesity causes cancer. More recent studies of this phenomenon have brought to light the fact that it is not the fat that causes the cancer but rather the high insulin levels that accompany the intake of high glycemic foods that obese people normally consume in large quantities. The ultimate solution to using sugar as a sweetener is to substitute stevia which is a white powder derived from a South American plant. A pinch of it produces the same sweetness as 3 tablespoons of sugar and it has 0 calories so it does not contribute to the production of fat or insulin spikes.

Stress and Cortisol

A major contributor to the formation of cancer are persistent negative feelings such as fear, despair and stress in general. If these emotional issues are chronic they can cause a continuous secretion of noradrenaline and cortisol.

These are the hormones that are secreted when we are frightened or upset. They serve a very useful purpose by providing us with the short-term energy we need to fight off or escape from a predator. However chronic stress in our lives tends to cause a constant low level seepage of cortisol into our systems. In preparation for any wounds we may receive these hormones increase our systemic levels of inflammation which unfortunately aids the growth of any cancer cells that may be present in our body. Systemic inflammation also greatly increases the chances of cardiovascular disease so that if cancer doesn't kill you then heart disease might.

Another thing that cortisol does is shut down all systems it considers to be useless. One of these "nonessentials" is the immune system. This is logical as the normal fight or flight situation lasts less than five minutes so that within 30 minutes the cortisol has been eliminated from our bodies and our immune system is back to functioning normally. Unfortunately when we are under continuous stress from relationship or work related issues it creates a steady drip of cortisol, which interferes with our immune system's ability to protect us for as long as we are upset. For this reason the elimination of stress from your life should be a number one priority.

X Radiation

One of the greatest advances in high-tech medical technology has been the CT scan. The problem is that each full body scan is the equivalent radiation exposure of 500 chest x-rays. There are 62 million CT scans of patients made every year in the United States for diagnostic purposes. Patients are usually not informed of the radiation doses that their bodies are absorbing during the scan. This is especially problematic for small children. The majority of radiation that people in advanced countries receive is from medical imaging. Studies estimate that CT scans alone are responsible for 30,000 cases of cancer each year. Unfortunately patients who've been scheduled for a CT scan are never told about the risks of cancer due to the radiation they will receive

Xenoestrogens

One of the functions of natural estrogen is to cause exponential cell growth during pregnancy. Environmental xenoestrogens are much stronger than natural estrogens and cause cancer cells to propagate rapidly. Unfortunately the effects of xenoestrogen exposure are cumulative over life. This is why xenoestrogens exacerbate the negative effects of natural estrogen especially in men. For 20 years it was thought that Testosterone replacement therapy for older men would cause prostate cancers to grow faster. It was later determined that testosterone was not causing the increased growth rate of prostate cancer. Their testosterone was being converted to estrogen by aromatase, which is produced in the fat cells. Since older men usually have higher fat percentages they had higher estrogen levels and it was actually their high levels of estrogen, which were causing their prostate cancers to grow faster.

The EPA estimates that 74 billion pounds of chemicals are being produced every day. Since it is virtually impossible for them to be disposed of in an environmentally friendly way, what is their final resting place after use? Most are chemically stable and do not degrade into harmless substances after use. Many are either Cariogenic or are Xenoestrogens, which cause cancer or cause hormone disruptions in our bodies.

Xenoestrogens are found in many household products. Researchers at the University of Cincinnati proved that bisphenol A (BPA) when heated diffuses into whatever substance it is in contact with. It is used as a plastic softener and is found in many products such as the linings of soda cans and food containers.

Another group of food additives that are highly carcinogenic are phosphates. The average person currently consumes 1,000mg of phosphates every day which is more than double the average dosage 25 years ago. Phosphates are found in nearly all carbonated beverages, fruit syrups, ice cream, frozen pizza and processed pastries.

All foods containing tri-calcium phosphate, disodium phosphate, phosphoric acid and calcium phosphate should be avoided. In a large research study of nearly 100,000 women it was found that the incidence of breast cancer was twice as high in those who consumed red meat seven or eight times a week as compared to those who consumed it less than three times a week. It was not necessarily the red meat that was causing the problem but rather the sodium nitrite and phosphates that were added as preservatives.

Another problem with meat products purchased at the supermarket is the amount of xenoestrogens that are absorbed from the plastic packaging that it is sold in. Another wildcard in studies of red meat causing cancer is that people who consume a lot of meat usually do not eat many anti-carcinogenic foods so it could be that aspect of their diet that is causing that group to have a higher rate of cancer rather than consumption of the meat itself.

Meat and dairy products as well as large fish account for 90% of human exposure to carcinogenic contaminants including pesticides and PCBs. Vegetables and fruit typically contain one hundredth the amount of contamination that is found in meat, tuna and milk. Pesticides are a major source of environmental toxins. The United States is the largest user at about 25% of total world production with Japan in second place. All of these chemicals and pesticides did not exist prior to 1940.

One of the most powerful xenoestrogens is atrazine which was used in household pesticides for more than 40 years in both the United States and Europe prior to being banned. The consumption of organic fruits and vegetables does make a tremendous difference in the levels of pesticides that accumulate within our bodies. Several research studies found that children who consumed organic foods had 1/4 the carcinogenic contamination of children whose diets was nonorganic.

List of xenoestrogens used in household products.

Name	Abbreviation	Use
4-Methylbenzylidene camphor	4-MBC	sunscreen lotions
methylparaben		preservative
ethylparaben		preservative
propylparaben		preservative
butylparaben		preservative
Benzophenone		Sunscreen lotions
Bisphenol A	BPA	Plastics
Phthalates		Plastics
DEHP		plasticizer for
Polybrominated biphenyl ethers	PBDE	flame retardants
Polychlorinated biphenyls	PCB	adhesives, paints
Erythrosine	Red No. 3	Food Color
Phenosulfothiazine		Red Dye
Butylated hydroxyanisole	BHA	food preservative
Pentachlorophenol		wood preservative
Atrazine		weed killer
Dieldrin		insecticide
Endosulfan		insecticide
Heptachlor		insecticide
Lindane		insecticide
hexachlorocyclohexane		insecticide
Methoxychlor		insecticide
Nonylphenol		emulsifiers
Propyl gallate		
Chlorine		
Ethinylestradiol		contraceptive

Cancer Relativity

Metalloestrogens		
Alkylphenol		detergents

8 CANCER CELL BIOLOGY

Medical dictionaries define cancer as an uncontrolled and abnormal growth of cells. Why are cancer cells uncontrollable by the normal regulatory mechanisms of the body? What are these normal controls and what causes them to fail? What turns an otherwise benign tumor into a cancerous one that spreads and takes over the body? What causes a benign tumor to suddenly become cancerous and dangerous to the person who has it?

Always remember that cancer cells have so mutated that they are crippled and frail to the point that almost anything will kill them on contact. If you can touch a cancer cell you can kill it within 5 days through the topical application of an ascorbic acid and water paste. I personally have used this particular therapy to cure at least four separate skin cancers that I have had. Unfortunately most hide out in the recesses of our bodies where they are impossible to get at.

Tumors are considered to be malignant when they suddenly acquire the ability to invade adjoining tissues and or release their cancerous cells into the bloodstream where they can travel to other parts of the body and begin new tumors. Cancer cannot occur in a persons body if it is functioning correctly simply because our immune systems are able to recognize and kill any cancerous cells that develop

Cancer cell metabolism

Most people believe that cancer just suddenly appears from out of nowhere due to exposure to carcinogens. The reality is that out of the trillions of cells that we have in our bodies a certain percentage are cancerous. A cluster of cancer cells must reach a level of detectability, which amounts to billions prior to them being reveled by cancer diagnostic tests. It normally takes years for them to proliferate to this extent.

A cancer that is suddenly detected by testing has in reality existed and grown for as much is 10 years before it was noticeable. Testing of the bodies of fatal accident victims for precancerous growths indicate that by the time we are 40 years old we have thousands of micro tumors throughout our bodies which are no threat to us because they lack the ability to generate their own blood vessels and therefore cannot grow larger than a few cells.

As has been stated previously cancer cells are "Obligate glucose feeders." Glucose is their only source of energy and it is metabolized through an anaerobic fermentation process rather than the normal cells oxygenation process. Although all carbs that we consume are converted into glucose the conversion of sugar is much more rapid and direct resulting in very high blood glucose levels. The Reduction of blood glucose levels is one of the primary ways we can reduce cancer's ability to survive in our bodies. The easiest way to accomplish this is to eliminate high glycemic carbs such as sugar, refined flour, and rice from our diets.

To understand why cancer cells must limit themselves to glucose as an energy source we need to learn how our cells mitochondria function. The primary task that our mitochondria perform is the utilization of energy sources other than glucose. Their secondary function is Apoptosis (Cell Death). So long as our blood glucose levels are high enough the mitochondria Use oxygen to break down the glucose to release energy for the cells use.

When insufficient glucose is present to support this process the fat in our fat cells goes through a conversion process and enters our bloodstream as ketones which the mitochondria can utilize the same as glucose to produce cellular energy. For this reason normal body cells are capable of utilizing multiple types of sugar for fuel but cancer cells can only utilize glucose because their mitochondria, if they even have any, are so damaged that they can not function properly. The results of a research study published in the October 2011 Journal of nutrition and metabolism indicated that increased levels of blood glucose caused cancer cell proliferation, inhibited apoptosis and encouraged angiogenesis.

The mitochondria Perform an occasional check of their cell to make sure that it has not mutated. If the cell's DNA has become corrupted the mitochondria initiates the process of apoptosis to kill it. When a cell's mitochondria become dysfunctional for whatever reason, the cell has no adult supervision. Now, if whatever damaged the mitochondria, radiation or carcinogens perhaps, also damaged the cells DNA enough that it has become cancerous, we have a problem.

Another characteristic of cancer cells is that because the fermentation process they use to produce energy is so inefficient they require 40% more energy input than a healthy cell to survive. Their inefficient conversion of glucose to energy through fermentation also produces a large quantity of acid as waste, which is excreted into the tissue surrounding them. An acidic saliva PH reading may be an indicator of cancer.

When a cell becomes cancerous it isn't necessarily a danger to us. Studies indicate that most people have tiny cancer cell clusters throughout their bodies consisting of only a few cells. In order to grow into tumors and spread they require the ability to generate their own circulatory system to acquire sufficient nutrients. They can then use these same blood vessels to transport cancer cells to other parts of the body where they can start new colonies of cells.

The easiest way to shut off a cancer's supply of fuel is to stop all intake of carbs and convert over to the use of ketones for your bodies energy source. Because a cancer cell is unable to generate a proper circulatory system within itself to carry away its' waste products it tends to accumulate a surrounding layer of its' own acidic waste which excludes our body's natural defenses from attacking the tumor. At the same time the tumor can release enzymes whose function is to dissolve the surrounding healthy cells and use them for fuel.

Some tumors can also cause the body to break down muscle protein into glucose through a process called glycogenesis. This is what causes end stage cancer patients to waste away and finally starve to death. When a tumor reaches this stage of self sufficiency about the only recourse is anti-angiogenic medications which terminate the tumor's ability to create and maintain its' system of blood vessels.

There are many different food based protocols for curing cancer all of which seem to be more or less effective. The one thing that they have in common is that none of them allow any high glycemic foods to be consumed. And especially not sugar. A recent Harvard research study has indicated that sugary carbonated drinks kill 200,000 people annually by causing cancer, diabetes and heart disease. Perhaps the first thing we should determine is what causes a cancer cell to come into existence and what specific characteristics does it need to threaten our continued existence.

When we are first borne our cells are new with very little contamination or damage. Their DNA strands have their full length of telomeres, which will protect their genetic code for the next 200 or so cell divisions. Unfortunately shortly after our birth our cells become the targets for every type of pathogen and carcinogenic pollutant that exists in our less than pristine environment. There comes a time usually around 30 years of age when the DNA of some of our 35 Trillion cells becomes sufficiently damaged that they can no longer function normally. Both the type of damage and the lack of functionality will vary greatly from cell to cell.

The continued survival of the new cancer cell at this point is to a great extent dependent upon the life style of the person in whose body it lives.

Mitochondria

More than 2 billion years ago when life was in its initial stages of development the atmosphere was quite different from what it is now. There was very little oxygen and the single celled organisms that existed at that time used anaerobic fermentation to produce their energy the same as cancer cells do today.

Unfortunately for them a new type of single celled organism was developing that could utilize carbon dioxide through primitive photosynthesis to produce its energy much the same as modern plants do. This new process used sunlight and the abundant supply of carbon dioxide to produce energy with oxygen as the waste product.

This process was much more efficient than the older fermentation process of producing energy that the other one celled life forms used. This gave the primitive cells that utilized it an exponentially greater ability to survive in a very competitive environment. This caused an increase in atmospheric oxygen, which caused a die off of most of the anaerobic organisms for whom oxygen was poisonous.

At some point one of the very large one celled organisms which relied on fermentation for its energy consumed some tiny bacteria that were the predecessors of our current day mitochondria but failed to digest them. This developed into a symbiotic relationship between the larger organism and the bacteria. The mitochondria were protected from predators and the larger cell in which they lived was able to utilize the energy produced by the smaller mitochondria living inside of it. This synergistic combination is what made multi-celled organisms possible.

Over the last two billion years the mitochondria have lost their independence from their host cells and much of their DNA has been incorporated into the cells DNA. The DNA which the mitochondria still have is almost identical to the DNA of simple bacteria which has a very different shape and structure then normal cell DNA. The mitochondria we currently have are completely dependent upon their host cells and have devolved from being an independent organism to being a cellular organelle that is completely subservient to its host cell and utilized solely for the production of the cell's energy. Without this symbiotic relationship the existence of large complex organisms would be impossible.

Our mitochondria generate chemical energy in the form of adenosine triphosphate (ATP) which is used to power the brain and neural system as well as our muscles. Our cells contain anywhere from two to two thousand mitochondria depending upon their energy needs. The mechanism by which this energy is produced is called the "electron transport chain", which consists of four protein complexes that work together to provide the necessary ingredients that fuel the fifth and final process, which occurs inside the mitochondria itself.

The first two processes of the four accepts negatively charged electrons which are generated by the digestion of food. These electrons are then transferred to the third process in the chain, which causes hydrogen protons to move across the inner mitochondrial membrane where they are joined by the electrons that were produced in processes one and two.

During this fourth process, which occurs inside the mitochondria, hydrogen and oxygen are combined to produce water. An electrical potential has now been created between the inner and outer sides of the mitochondrial membrane which is used by the fifth process within the mitochondria to create more than 30 ATP molecules which are then used by the cell for its' energy needs.

Because of its bacterial origins mitochondrial DNA is very different from the DNA contained in our cell nuclei. It has a circular shape reminiscent of its bacterial origins and unlike the single strand of DNA contained in a cell's nucleus, mitochondria can have many copies of their DNA. Another difference is that we inherit our cellular DNA equally from both of our parents. Our mitochondrial DNA on the other hand is 100% maternal in origin with none of it coming from our fathers.

Because mitochondria have multiple sets of their DNA the case may arise where some of the DNA sets are damaged and contain mutations. If this is the case how does the mitochondria Know which set of DNA is correct and usable and which ones are mutations and should not be utilized. It is a simple case of percentages the mitochondria will choose the DNA set that is most prevalent, the one it was born with. When the percentage of mutated DNA sets becomes greater than 50% the mitochondria will start to show signs of dysfunction.

As our cells age so do their mitochondria. Could this be why historically cancer has always been an affliction of old age? Could the reason for the increase in incidents of cancer in young people be an indication of mitochondrial DNA damage caused by environmental factors and poor nutrition? Perhaps the causal mechanism is based on time versus concentration. Perhaps it is a slow but inevitable process which is based on level of exposure over a certain period of time.

Our mitochondria have another function which is almost as important as their ability to provide us with our energy to survive. They have the power of life and death for the cell they currently inhabit. If they determine that either their own or their host cell's DNA has mutated they will kill the cell through a process called apoptosis. This is our body's first line of defense against cancer cell formation. Unfortunately there are trillions of cells in our bodies and the odds are that a few of these cells will have mitochondria which are damaged in such a way that they will fail to kill their cell if it becomes cancerous.

9 INFLAMMATION AND CANCER

Persons who are obese have a 40% higher rate of cancer. Therefore obesity obviously causes cancer! Or maybe it is cancer that causes obesity. Cause and effect relationships are quite often a chore to sort out. When two conditions coexist never fall into the trap of believing that one must be the cause and the other the effect. Quite often they are both the effects of an unspecified cause. So let me be very specific. Sugar and other high glycemic index foods are the main contributor to both conditions.

The process of storing and later utilizing fat for energy is highly inflammatory, which causes the formation of a large number of free radicals and oxidants. For this reason it is better if we strictly limit our consumption of carbohydrates and sugars to keep this process in check. Insulin which is involved in the conversion and transport of fatty acids into fat cells for storage is also extremely inflammatory. High glycemic foods because of the rapidity with which they raise our blood sugar and insulin levels are highly inflammatory as well. I believe that one of the reasons diabetics have a much higher incidence of cancer is that over dosing of insulin creates a very high level of inflammation for extended periods of time.

Cancer cells are "Obligate Glucose Feeders". This means that glucose is the only energy source that they are capable of utilizing. Add to this the fact that cancer cells require 40% more energy to survive than normal cells and it becomes obvious that the consumption of large amounts of sugar and other foods that are quickly converted to sugar is not a good survival strategy. Refined sugar produces and maintains this high blood glucose level, which cancer cells desperately need. It is also the worst systemic inflammatory that we consume and there is growing evidence that inflammation of the arterial walls is what causes cholesterol to adhere to them. Sugar therefore is trying to kill us in three different ways:

1. By making us obese.

2. By providing the only food source that cancer cells can utilize.

3. By inflaming our arteries, which allows cholesterol to adhere forming plaque deposits.

There are many different types of cancer prevention diets some are low-fat plant based diets others are low carb high fat diets. The common denominator in all of these successful cancer prevention diets is that they all greatly reduce or eliminate sugar. So basically you can utilize whatever type of diet that conforms to your ideology so long as it is sugar free. I suggest that you simply substitute powdered Stevia for the sugar and have the best of both worlds.

10 CONVENTIONAL CANCER TREATMENTS

"One of the first duties of the physician is to educate the masses not to take medicine."

Sir William Osler, 1849-1919 Medical Historian

"Half of the modern drugs could well be thrownout of the window, except that the birds might eat them."

Dr. M. H. Fischer

None of the medical experts seem to be able to agree on what cancer is let alone how to cure it. If they find a lump and excise it you will hear the most ubiquitous lie in cancer treatment "I think we got it all." It's a lie because that wasn't the cancer that they removed only a local manifestation of its more systemic presence. During the Victorian era cancer was so rare that it was considered an oddity. The average Victorian got plenty of exercise by walking 10 miles per day and consumed healthy organic produce. During that era only 1 in 5,000 developed cancer during their lifetimes. Today the cancer rate is approaching 1 in 2. Now that's progress!

There are only three FDA approved treatments for cancer. They are surgery, chemotherapy and radiation. Oncology's definition of a successful treatment is if the patient manages to survive for five more years. Now, take a look at the chart on the next page and tell me how successful chemotherapy is by mainstream medicine's own definition of success!

Type of Malignancy	No. of Patients	No. of 5 year Survivors	% of 5 year Survivors
Head and neck	2486	63	2.5
Esophagus	1003	54	4.8
Stomach	1904	13	0.7
Colon	7243	128	1.8
Rectum	4036	218	5.4
Pancreas	1728	0	0.0
Lung	7792	118	1.5
Soft tissue sarcoma	665	0	0.0
Melanoma of Skin	7811	0	0.0
Breast	10661	164	1.5
Uterus	1399	0	0.0
Cervix	867	104	12
Ovary	1207	105	8.7
Prostate	9869	0	0.0
Testis	529	221	41.8
Bladder	2802	0	0.0
2802 Kidney	2176	0	0.0
Brain	1116	55	4.9
Unknown primary site	3161	0	0.0
Non-Hodgkin's lymphoma	3145	331	10.5
Hodgkin's disease	341	122	35.8
Multiple myeloma	1023	0	0.0
Total	72,903	1690	2.3%

You can find the complete research paper by plugging this locator code into Google.

Clinical Oncology (2004) 16: 549e560 doi:10.1016/j.clon.2004.06.007

With the possible exception of Hodgkin's disease and testicular cancer you would get a better five-year survival rate using a placebo! I'm not exaggerating, it's been tested. In most cases placebos do work better than chemotherapy. The five-year survival statistics for radiation therapy are about the same. No matter how focused the radiation beam is some surrounding healthy cells will be damaged to the point that they will become cancerous themselves within a few years.

Cancer patients instinctively do not want to do chemo but everyone tells them they have to. Initially there is success and their physician tells them that they are in remission but after a few months it's back. There is speculation that chemo can make the cancer spread and become more aggressive. The national toxicology board lists many of the chemo drugs as carcinogens.

The Long-term success rate of both chemotherapy and radiation is 2.5-5%. When an oncologist says that his treatment was successful what he means is that the patient managed to survive for five years before dying. Numerous studies have conclusively demonstrated that people who refuse to be treated for their cancer survive an average of 12 years. According to research studies performed in Scotland by Dr. Ewan Cameron and Linus Pauling, vitamin C therapy allowed cancer patients to survive six times longer on average than chemotherapy patients. They also enjoyed a better quality of life because the vitamin C therapy strengthened their immune systems instead of weakening them.

If someone was marketing an alternative treatment for cancer and they told their perspective patients that they would have to spend at least a year watching their hair fall out and puking into the toilet all for a 2.5% probability that they would manage to live 5 more years. and that it would only cost them $150,000 everyone would laugh, call him a "Quack rip-off artist" and walk away shaking their heads. When the medical establishment offers a cancer patient the same deal he signs up. Such is the power of a lifetime of propaganda.

Although it is claimed that radiation therapy does not adversely affect the normal tissue surrounding a tumor many breast cancer victims who receive radiation therapy go on to develop lung cancer in later years. (Med Oncol, 1994; 11: 121–5). One study has shown that lung cancer patients who receive radiation therapy have a 20% greater chance of death. (Cochrane Database Syst Rev, 2003; 1: CD002142). The drugs used in chemotherapy are designed to kill any cells that have high proliferation rates regardless of whether they are cancerous or not.

Chemotherapy when used in conjunction with radiation therapy was shown to have no desirable effect on the survival rates of the cancer patients in this study. (JAMA, 1991; 265: 391–5). Another cancer specialist did a detailed study of all data he could find on chemotherapy cure rates in cases of advanced cancer. His conclusion was the same as the other study that chemo drugs do not prolong survival. (Biomed Pharmacother, 1992; 46: 439–52)

Illness of any kind is the body's check engine light. It indicates that something is wrong with the body systemically. You can fix it by break the warning light and then when the engine begins to make noises you can turn up your stereo. When you begin to hear it over the stereo... well then you obviously need to install a more powerful amplifier. This is called treating the symptom instead of the disease. Physicians are incredibly good at this. There is a medication for everything but a cure for nothing.

46% of cancer patients die of malnutrition. The other most common causes of cancer patient deaths are opportunistic infections such as pneumonia or multi organ failure caused by system overload. Cancer usually doesn't kill patients directly, they usually die of the secondary health problems caused by the chemo. A person needs to be weak and sick in the first place for cancer to develop then we do everything possible during their treatment to make them weaker and sicker.

How Conventional treatment is made to look good

The success of surgery is inversely proportionate to the malignancy of the tumor that they are removing. In other words tumors that are not malignant and pose no real threat can be removed very successfully. However tumors that are seriously malignant and contain Cancer cells quite often are declared inoperable thereby generating no averse data for conventional treatment.

When a cancer patient dies of infection it is because the chemotherapy destroyed his immune system to the point where he could not fight off the infection. The medical community then records the cause of death as infection rather than the chemotherapy itself.

If the statistical average for breast cancer is two women out of every hundred and a drug company conducts a research study on a group of 100 women and at the end of that study only one of them developed breast cancer the company claims that its drug caused a 50% reduction in the cancer rate. When in reality it was only a 1% reduction. The 50% reduction is the relative benefit and the 1% is the absolute benefit.

Obviously the 50% figure is much more impressive than the other and is the one the drug company will use to sell their product. Another drug company trial reported that the drug tamoxifen produced a 50% decrease in the rate of breast cancer. The relative benefit was 50% the absolute benefit was 1.5 people out of 100. Less than a Placebo. Unfortunately most of the oncologists who are treating patient's believe the pharmaceutical company's numbers.

The majority of oncologists state that neither they or anyone in their families would ever undergo either radiation or chemotherapy if they were diagnosed with cancer because they believe it to be ineffective and overly toxic. Each year the cancer death rate increases in spite of the billions of dollars spent on conventional cancer treatments and the billions of dollars of research that goes into trying to cure it.

When a cancer is surgically removed from a patient damage is done not only to the tissue surrounding the tumor but also to its blood supply network. This requires the body to rebuild that vascular system where the incision was made and a part of this process is regeneration of new blood vessels, which the remaining cells of the cancer, which were left behind can tap into and utilize for their own blood supply. This might be why cancerous growths seem to spread and become more active after surgical removal of the main tumor.

11 SPONTANEOUS REGRESSION OF CANCER

Most oncologist today claim that the human body has no natural cancer fighting ability and do not believe in spontaneous regression of cancers even though thousands of cases have been reported. They always claim that it was either a misdiagnosis and the patient did not really have cancer in the first place or if the patient received any kind of conventional treatment, no matter how little, it is claimed that that small amount of conventional treatment was what actually cured the cancer. Norwegian researchers have determined that if left completely untreated at least 20% of breast cancer cases spontaneously regress. (Arch Intern Med, 2008; 168: 2311–6)

Another study indicated that 25% of lymphoma patients who did not receive treatment experienced spontaneous regression (N Engl J Med, 1984; 311: 1471–5). Cases of spontaneous regression seem to be much more prevalent in children than adults. All of this brings up the possibility that all of us come down with cancer but that for two out of three spontaneous regression occurs and those cancers never give any indication of their presence before they disappear. Considering that the five-year cure rate for conventional cancer treatments is only a little over 2% it would seem that just leaving cancers alone even without any kind of nutritional intervention gives 10 times the cure rate as radiation, surgery and chemotherapy.

During the 1980s a couple of researchers at the Erasmus University in Rotterdam decided to do a metadata study to determine the veracity of this assertion. They only included cases where the original diagnosis of cancer prior to treatment or non-treatment was unassailable. After a year and a half of research which was confined only to their small region of Holland they found seven cases of spontaneous regression of cancer that could not be disputed.

Many studies have been performed which indicate that cancer patients who take a proactive stance and educate themselves concerning cancer and try to control their weight, consume foods that are anti-carcinogenic, stop consuming foods that have been proven to promote cancer and received plenty of exercise live three times longer than patients who don't. Their quality of life is also improved.

Fever is our body's way of killing pathogens within our bodies. It could well be that many of the spontaneous regression cases are caused by elevated body temperatures from fever. In 1866 Prof. Busch deliberately infected a cancer patient with live streptococcus bacteria. This produced a high fever in the patient followed by spontaneous regression from the cancer. This procedure has been used by many different physicians ever since up until the early 60s when the FDA made the use of it illegal.

Curiously enough during the 1960s various pharmaceutical companies developed and marketed the same fever inducing pathogens with mixed success. However since the same patients were receiving chemotherapy it could well be that the chemotherapy reduce the effectiveness of their immune systems to the point that in many cases it rendered the fever therapy ineffective. In one study it was found that in subjects who had three or four infections of more than 38°C the frequency of melanoma fell by 40%. (Melanoma Res, 1999; 9: 511–9)

One of the most famous cases of spontaneous regression of cancer occurred by accident when Zheng Cui a professor of biology at Wake Forest University was in the process of infecting mice with sarcoma cancer cells which grew so aggressively that their numbers doubled every 12 hours. He was performing the routine procedure of injecting large quantities of these cancer cells into the abdominal cavities of mice. He would then extract the fluids that built up within the mice and use it for his experiments.

None of the mice ever survived more than one month. There was however one exception in that mouse number six seemed to be completely immune to the cancer cell injections and his body managed to destroy every cancer cell that was injected into him. Because of this puzzling immunity he was singled out to be injected with doses of cancer cells that were 1000 times greater than normal fatal doses all of which he successfully defeated and went on to live eight times longer than any of the other mice and at the same time experiencing no ill effects.

They decided to breed him to other normal female mice with the result that half of their resulting offspring also demonstrated the same immunity to cancer as their father. These special mice are now extensively used in the testing of genetically caused cancer regression.

Prof. Zheng Cui later made an additional accidental discovery. When he returned to the laboratory after a seven month sabbatical he found that all of the mice involved in his studies were symptomatic for the cancer cell injections and no longer seemed to be immune. He was very despondent and discontinued his study of the mice for a month. Upon finally returning to the lab and checking on the mice he discovered that they were now cancer free and completely normal.

He eventually figured out that at approximately 6 months of age or the equivalent of 50 years for humans their immune systems were temporarily weakened and the cancer started to take hold but approximately 2 weeks later the equivalent of two years in human lifespan the tumor's presence activated the immune system which then aggressively attacked and killed off the cancer cells. This phenomenon has been observed in humans as well. It could be that there is up to a two year delay before our immune system finally classifies the growth as cancerous and begins to kill it.

12 CANCER TREATMENTS THAT ALTER BODY PH

In 1931 Dr. Otto Warburg received the Nobel Prize for medical research into the causes of cancerous growths. Until recently those discoveries have been ignored by the medical establishment and are only recently being accepted as the correct description of the cause for cancer cell development. One of Dr. Warburg's cancer cell experiments consisted of lowering the oxygen levels of normal cells by 35% for 48 hours, these normal tissue cells became cancerous and remained cancerous even after the level of oxygen was returned to normal.

It was also determined that they were now utilizing the fermentation (Glycolysis) of blood sugars to produce their energy rather than the normal oxygen driven metabolic process of healthy cells. Another one of his experiments demonstrated that cancer cells cannot tolerate the normal alkaline environment of the body. Cancer cells can only thrive in an environment with a very low acidic PH. A normal cell's natural environment is alkaline and high in oxygen whereas cancer cells prefer an environment that is acidic and completely deprived of oxygen.

Dr. Warburg said it best during a lecture to a meeting of Nobel laureates in Lindau Germany on June 30, 1966 "From the standpoint of the physics and chemistry of life, this difference between normal and cancer cells is so great that one can scarcely imagine a greater difference. Oxygen gas, the donor of energy in plants and animals, is dethroned in cancer cells, and replaced by an energy-yielding reaction of the lowest living forms, namely, a fermentation of glucose, The early history of life on our planet indicates that life existed on Earth before the atmosphere contained free oxygen gas, The living cells must therefore have been fermenting cells and, as fossils show, they were undifferentiated single cells.

Only when free oxygen appeared in the atmosphere some two billion years ago did the higher development of life set in to produce the plant and animal kingdoms from the fermenting, undifferentiated single cells. The reverse process, the de-differentiation of life, takes place in cancer development. The highly differentiated cells are transformed into non-oxygen breathing fermenting cells, which have lost all their body functions and retain only the now useless property of growth. What remains are growing machines that destroy the body in which they grow."

Dr. Warburg's observations and experiments have recently been verified using modern medical research equipment and he is finally beginning to receive the credit that he is due. (Cancer Res, 2005; 65: 613–21). (Nat Rev Cancer, 2004; 4: 891–9) (Cancer Res, 2002; 62: 6674–81) (Proc Natl Acad Sci USA, 2005; 102: 5992–7) (Curr Opin Clin Nutr Metab Care, 2006; 9: 339–45) Current research indicates that people who receive sufficient exercise to maintain the oxygenation of their body tissues reduce their chances of cancer by 50%.

One of the main reasons for the ever increasing amount of cancer is the systemic level of acid within our bodies due to our modern diet which is high in processed carbohydrates. Consumption of green vegetables, fresh fruits and spices have fallen to the lowest levels in history while our consumption of artificial processed foods containing large amounts of high fructose corn syrup have increased exponentially. Rather than trying to eradicate cancer cells once they have grown and multiplied it would be far better to maintain an environment within our bodies that is not conducive to the formation of cancer cells in the first place. Unfortunately nearly 100% of current medical research involves trying to cure cancers after they have metastasized and become a systemic problem.

If we allow an acidic condition to exist within our bodies for an extended period of time it provides an environment in which cancer cells can reproduce and thrive. Research has demonstrated that terminal cancer patients often have levels of acidity much greater than a normal healthy person and as little as 50% of the oxygenation. The opposite is also true. When a persons body PH is alkaline (normal is 7.5 on the PH scale) it favors normal aerobic energy production through the utilization of oxygen. Our bodies require an alkaline pH in order to optimize the utilization of oxygen for the normal production of energy.

This is why exercise is so important. It increases the efficiency of oxygen transport within our bodies leading to an alkaline body PH. Then because the body is alkaline it is better able to utilize the oxygen it receives. Another downside to a highly acidic condition is that it causes the person to be fatigued because our cells cannot take up and convert oxygen to energy as efficiently as when they have an alkaline environment to operate in. Often to the point of depression developing. The depression and anxiety can then trigger the cortisol axis which will shut down the immune system to conserve energy and allow cancer cells to flourish.

If our cells become deprived of oxygen for whatever reason it can cause an increase in the acidity of cells within the area were oxygen deprivation occurs. This lack of oxygen and acidic pH work together to produce an environment that is very conducive for the growth of cancer cells. The reason that all of this works for the cancer cell even though it is far less efficient than normal cell respiration. Is that by separating and isolating its' metabolic processes from the rest of the body it can avoid attacks by our immune system because our white blood cells are incapable of penetrating the coating of acid that covers cancer cells.

This acidic coating results from the inefficient fermentation process that produces the acid as a waste product which is then excreted to the outside of the cancer cell's membrane and prevents white blood cells from recognizing and attacking the cancer cell.

It is a good idea to occasionally test our systemic PH level to make sure that it is in the correct range. By being aware of our bodies pH we will be able to maintain it at the proper level so that cancers if they currently exist will be killed and new ones kept from being created. The most effective way to control our body's PH is by consuming foods that produce an alkaline condition instead of ones that contribute to an acidic condition within our bodies. At a pH level of 7.5 cancer cells become dormant while a systemic PH of 8.5 will cause cancer cells to die and at the same time will be beneficial for healthy cells.

If we want to limit the ability of cancer cells to exist within our bodies the first thing we need to do is determine what types of foods we should be eating to promote an alkaline environment within our bodies that will prevent that formation. This means that we should eat foods that are rich in alkaline minerals such as magnesium potassium and calcium along with the usual antioxidants and vitamins.

At its most basic level what is needed with few exceptions is to increase the amount of food with a pH higher than seven that we consume and decrease the amount of foods that we consume that have a pH lower than seven. The exception to this rule is that any type of fruit is beneficial as a cancer preventative even if it is acidic. Your first line of defense against having an acidic condition is aerobic exercise rather than supplementation.

Self testing your PH is very simple. All you need are PH test strips to test the pH of your saliva. You should wait about two hours after eating. Touch the end of the pH strip to your tongue coating the colored squares on its' end with your saliva and compare it to the color chart on the side of the container the pH strips came in. If you're saliva gives an acid indication wait a couple of hours and repeat the test to make sure that no anomalies crept into the testing that caused a false positive indication. While children tend to have a very healthy pH a large percentage of adults have a pH of 6.5 or lower which reflects the low intake of calcium, magnesium and other alkaline minerals and or lack of exercise.

All of this might lead us to the conclusion that we should eliminate all fruits and vegetables from our diet which are acidic. This however is not the case because many of the fruits and vegetables which are prohibited by the people who promote this type of anti-cancer alkaline therapy have been proven to be extremely anti-carcinogenic.

Research studies have proven that tomatoes, most berries including strawberries, and ascorbic acid to name a few are highly anti-angiogenic and prevent cancers from developing their own blood vessel system thereby reducing tumor size exponentially and preventing new tumors from growing beyond the size of a pinpoint.

Coffee is also acidic but research studies have proven that 4 cups a day will reduce your susceptibility to cancer by 40%. Coffee enemas are extremely beneficial for proper liver function, which is essential for proper operation of our immune systems. So we must be careful when considering a particular regime to cure cancer and instead of blindly eliminating everything from our diet that is proscribed by that particular discipline we need to always compare successful treatments against each other to make certain that all variables have been taken into account so that we can optimize our treatment.

One of the first things we can safely eliminate from our diet is all forms of carbonated beverages because of their very high acid content and their having no health benefits whatsoever. Because of the depleted condition of the soil in which most of our produce is grown most everyone who does not supplement their diet with minerals and vitamins will find that they are sufficiently deficient that their immune systems are seriously impaired.

Here is a list of minerals which have very high pH values and therefore are exceptionally beneficial in our fight against cancer. Calcium, magnesium and potassium are the three most critical ones to consume in sufficient quantities because of the thousands of critical biological processes that they support. Bicarbonate of soda is most commonly recommended for lowering PH. I do not recommend using it because unlike the other five minerals it has no secondary health benefits and can become a health hazard if too much is consumed. Magnesium, Calcium and Potassium on the other hand are essential nutrients that support thousands of biological processes within our bodies.

Bicarbonate of soda	PH 14
Calcium	PH 12
Cesium	PH 14
Magnesium	PH 9
Potassium	PH 14
Selenium	PH 9

The proper ratio of calcium to magnesium

The ideal ratio of calcium to magnesium seems to be about 2:1. In order to calculate your correct dosage of supplemental magnesium you will first need to determine your approximate daily intake of calcium. If you do not consume a significant amount of dairy products you can safely supplement 1000 mg of calcium and 500 mg of magnesium. However if you consume a large quantity of dairy products such as cheese and milk you will need to calculate the approximate calcium that you are receiving from them and subtract that from the 1000 mg of calcium supplementation.

The reason for this is that excessive calcium in our systems that is not utilized by biological processes can form kidney stones as well as plaque on the inside of our arteries. Dosages over 500 mg of magnesium on the other hand will usually cause diarrhea in most people. These parameters need to be tailored to the individual so you will have to experiment and come up with a ratio that seems to work best for you.

A proper level of magnesium is vital for the proper utilization of calcium as well as vitamin D by our bodies. Magnesium converts vitamin D into its active form at which point it can assist with the proper absorption of calcium into our bones. Magnesium also stimulates the production of the hormone calcitonin which is utilized by our bodies to draw calcium deposits from our blood and soft tissues moving them back into our bones where they belong.

This lowers the probability of osteoporosis as well as arthritis, heart attack and the formation of kidney and gallstones. There is growing evidence that systemic inflammation of our vascular system is what actually causes cholesterol and calcium to form plaque on their interiors. So making sure that 100% of the calcium that we consume is properly utilized is essential not only for the health of our bones but our cardiovascular system as well.

Magnesium gluconate is much more readily absorbed by our heart muscle cells which require large quantities of it for proper function so it would probably be best to use that particular type of magnesium. Insufficient magnesium in our diets also contributes to inflammation and oxidation. Potassium is important because it regulates proper heart rhythm, blood pressure, hydration, digestion and muscle cell contraction.

Diet is generally the single greatest determinant of body pH as well as oxygenation levels. Acidosis is further aggravated by a lack of critical minerals. Most effective cancer cures somehow involve adjusting the body's pH into the ideal alkaline state whether that is their intention or not. In an alkaline state, human blood is rich in oxygen. Blood saturated with oxygen is typically poisonous to cancer cells. Cancer cells are fragile and easy to kill through the introduction of various nutrients and minerals which create an environment within our bodies that is not conducive to supporting them.

Candida fungus

The latest person to propose an alternative theory to cure cancer was Dr. Tullio Simoncini. An Italian oncologist who suggested that cancer is not a genetic condition but is caused by the aggression of a fungus called Candida Albicans. For this reason he treats cancer with bicarbonate of soda which is very effective at killing fungus. He found it very interesting that all tumors behave in the same way even though their cells are different from one another so he started looking for a common denominator that would account for all of them.

He found that all cancer growths are white and that the Candida fungus is always present during autopsies of cancer victims as well. The medical establishment simply considers it to be an opportunistic infection by the fungus. Normally our immune systems keep this fungus under control and do not allow it to establish colonies within our bodies. Dr. Simoncini believes that the formation of the tumor is the body's way of trying to isolate and reject the fungus infection and that the only solution to this rampant infection by the candida is to reinforce the immune system so that it's better able to keep this fungus under control.

If a person is given chemotherapy instead it only increases the virulence of the fungus attack and accelerates its' growth. To try and prove his theory the doctor began treating cancer with bicarbonate of soda. He then presented his findings to the Italian medical establishment for review and testing. For his efforts he was disciplined and lost his medical license. This is unfortunate since even thousand-year-old books of Indian medical cures recommend bicarbonate of soda as a cure for cancer. Dr. Simoncini used the bicarbonate of soda because it was the only antifungal agent he knew of that could be ingested. His actual recommendation is to develop standard prescription antifungal medications that can be taken in sequentially stronger doses to kill the systemic fungus.

Thoughts:

Baking soda is a standard procedure for treating a person with an acidic PH. It could well be that his theory about the origin of cancer is incorrect but that his cure of using bicarbonate of soda to try and kill the fungus actually succeeded in raising his patients alkalinity level thereby arresting the development of their cancers.

Conclusions

1. Oxygenation of our bodies must be maintained through exercise as well as proper nutrition.

2. Our body fluids must be maintained at a pH of 7.5 or higher.

3. High levels of hemoglobin should be maintained in order to transport oxygen more efficiently.

4. The difference between a healthy body cell and a cancerous one is enormous. These differences can be utilized to our advantage for both prevention and treatment of cancers.

13 ANTI-ANGIOGENESIS

Angiogenesis is the process that our bodies use to grow blood vessels of which the human body has 60,000 miles. An interesting characteristic of blood vessels is that they can adapt to whatever type of tissue they grow in. For example in the liver they adapt themselves to the detoxification of blood, in the lungs to the exchange of gases. In muscle they are spiral shaped so that muscle contraction will not restrict circulation. Blood vessels do not normally propagate in adults. However many we are born with are all that we will have with the exception of wound repair.

Our bodies have the ability to regulate the formation of new blood vessels at any given time and location by the release of stimulators and inhibitors of angiogenesis. If we need blood vessels in a specific area to heal a wound the body can accomplish this by releasing angiogenic factors that act to stimulate the production of new blood vessels. If later, those vessels are no longer needed the body releases inhibitors of angiogenesis that reduce the quantity back to the baseline. After an injury our bodies release angiogenic stimulators in the damaged area that promote the growth of new blood vessels to replace the ones lost due to the injury. Allowing the new tissue that is being formed to receive an adequate blood supply.

Various diseases are able to exploit defects in this system so that the body can't reduce the number of extra blood vessels or is incapable of growing enough new ones in a location where they are needed. In these situations angiogenesis is said to be out of balance and when this occurs a disease is the result. For example insufficient angiogenesis leads to wounds that don't heal, legs without circulation and nerve damage. Cancer is often able to encourage and exploit excessive angiogenesis. In total there are more than 70 major diseases, which though they seem to be different have abnormal angiogenesis in common. If we can control angiogenesis we can then use it to control not only these diseases but cancer as well.

The main difference between a successful metastatic cancer that grows and spreads and one that remains microscopic is its' ability to encourage and then utilize angiogenesis to produce its' own blood vessels and then use them to bring nutrients to it as well as to remove waste products. All cancers start out as a small microscopic nest of cells that can only grow to a maximum of one half cubic millimeter in size because they don't have a blood supply to provide enough nutrients. Autopsy studies indicate that about 40% of women and 50% of men have these tiny cancer clusters. However without a blood supply these cancers will never become dangerous or even detectable and will eventually be eliminated by our immune system.

When the body is working properly its' ability to balance angiogenesis prevents blood vessels from feeding cancer and this is one of our most important defense mechanisms against it. If however a cancer can simulate an injury by producing inflammation in the area surrounding it the body can be tricked into the releasing the angiogenic factors in that area. The body will then respond by growing capillaries in the area that it thinks is damaged because of the inflammation. The tumor can then grow exponentially and this is how a cancer goes from harmless to deadly.

There are two ways to control undesirable angiogenesis. One is through prescription medications some of which are very effective and infinitely less harmful than chemotherapy. The other is by the consumption of various fruits and vegetables whose efficacy has been proven in research studies and that are often as effective as the prescription medications at controlling angiogenesis.

Angiostatin is the anti-angiogenic factor that our bodies release to inhibit the growth of new blood vessels. Today there are drugs which mimic the effects of Angiostatin and have proven very effective in shrinking the size of existing tumors by interfering with their ability to induce blood vessel growth. Angiostatin only inhibits the propagation of very fast growing capillaries and does not cause any damage to existing branches of the blood system. Cancer is a product of its ability to mimic our bodies responses to injury through the creation of inflammation in the area surrounding it and taking advantage of our body's natural response of releasing angiogenic factors in that area because it assumes that there has been tissue damage that requires revascularization.

This causes the creation of new capillary systems within the cancerous areas through angiogenesis. Anything that we can do to fight inflammation within our bodies helps prevent inappropriate angiogenesis. Continually oxygenating our bodies through daily exercise to keep our body's PH alkaline and supporting our overworked immune systems will exponentially improve our chances of staying cancer free throughout our lives.

Berries of most any type contain ellagic acid and studies have shown that normal dietary doses of berries especially raspberries and strawberries significantly slow the growth of tumors in mice. This fact is well known by nearly every cancer research center and pharmaceutical company but because a naturally occurring fruit or vegetable is not patentable there is no profit to be made. Which of course doesn't concern us because all we have to do is add berries to our daily diet to gain this protection. Not only does ellagic acid help prevent angiogenesis but it also blocks the effects of environmental toxins that damage our DNA.

Cranberries, cinnamon, unsweetened dark chocolate, cherries and blueberries all contain anthocyanidins and proanthocyanidins molecules that have been proven to force cancer cells to commit suicide (apoptosis). Breast cancer patients who consumed raspberries experienced a 50% reduction in tumors and polyps over their peers who received no raspberries in their diet. Nectarines, plums and peaches also provide the same protective nutrients as the berries. (Cancer Prevention Research 187 (2009). DOI: doi: 10.1158/1940-

6207.CAPR-08-0226)

The prescription medication Gleevec introduced in 2001 helps prevent angiogenesis in cancer tumors and has been shown to be quite effective. There are however many herbs and spices which are equally effective in preventing the proliferation of capillaries within cancer tumors. Spices such as basil, thyme, oregano, rosemary, mint and marjoram have a high concentration of Terpene fatty acids which is what makes them so fragrant. These herbs have both anti-angiogenic and apoptotic properties when they come in contact with cancer cells. Parsley and celery both contain apigenine which has been shown to inhibit the generation of tumor supporting capillaries equally well as the prescription drug Gleevec.

Anti-angiogenic substances found in fruits and vegetables are highly synergistic. Mice with breast cancer who were fed only one natural anti-carcinogenic experienced a 50% lower probability of that cancer getting out of control. However when fed three or more different varieties of natural cancer inhibitors they had a 90% chance of their cancer going into remission. (Cancer Research 67, no. 2 (2007): 836-43)

This synergy is probably caused by each fruit or vegetable containing a slightly different anti-carcinogen, each of which attacks the cancer cells from a slightly different direction therefore providing greater efficacy. The study cited above also indicates that tomatoes and broccoli are very synergistic in this manner when they are consumed during the same meal.

This is one of the things that drives the pharmaceutical companies crazy. If they could just isolate one chemical from one of these natural anti-carcinogenic sources they might be able to patent it. Unfortunately they all need to be consumed as a whole thereby eliminating any possibility of profit being made off of any research into them. Thus far no research study has evaluated the synergistic affects of the combination of all of the known anti-carcinogenic foods and spices. You however can perform the study yourself at almost no expense and potentially tremendous health benefits. All that you need to do is include all the following in your weekly meal plans and you don't even need to be that consistent about it.

Drink 4 cups of green tea and or 4 cups of good light roasted coffee per day.

Reduce your intake of Omega-6 and increase your intake of omega-3 fatty acids.

Use spices, especially turmeric.

Use herbs when you cook as they were meant to be used. (Large amounts and lots of different types.)

Broccoli and tomatoes together at least three times a week.

Extra virgin olive oil and garlic whenever possible.

Onions, leeks, chives and green onions. Parsley and cilantro as well.

Berries, peaches, apricots, nectarines and bell peppers.

All of these particular food items are well represented in a number of cuisines such as Thai, Indian, Chinese and Mediterranean. These are the most healthy anti cancer and heart healthy cuisines in the world for a reason.

There's been much discussion concerning the proper way to prepare foods for consumption without reducing their anti-carcinogenic effects because of heating. A couple of research studies have been done concerning this and have found that with the exception of frying, broiling and grilling at high temperatures very little harm is done to the cancer fighting nutrients that these foods contain.

Cruciform vegetables such as broccoli, brussels sprouts and cauliflower should be steamed at low temperature rather than boiled so that they retain their nutritional value. Freezing foods does not interfere with the anticancer ingredients that they contain as well. The only exception is seafood, which should be steamed rather than grilled or fried to maintain the quality of the Omega-3 fatty acids that it contains. (Plant Foods for Human Nutrition 63, no. 2 (June 2008): 47-52)

William Li, head of the Angiogenesis Foundation has done some very interesting research into both pharmacological and natural ways to prevent unwanted angiogenesis. In one study that he conducted on a group of 600 dogs with terminal cancer he achieved a 60% cure rate using the standard anti-angiogenic medications. Other research trials of these new drugs which have been available since 2004 indicate that they provide a 70% to 100% improvement in survival for people with kidney, myeloma, colorectal and gastrointestinal tumors over the usual radiation, chemo and surgical treatments.

Dr. Li has compiled a list of fruits and vegetables that his research facility has proven to be nearly as effective as the anti-angiogenic pharmaceuticals. What is interesting is that most of them have been promoted as anti-carcinogenic and good for our health in general for hundreds of years.

Plants with Anti-angiogenic and Anti-inflammatory Properties

Common Name	Latin Name	Action
Aloe Vera	Aloe Vera	Anti-inflammatory
Apples		Anti-angiogenic
Artichokes		Anti-angiogenic
Asian pine	Camellia Sinensis	Anti-inflammatory
Blackberries		Anti-angiogenic
Blueberries		Anti-angiogenic

Bok Choy		Anti-angiogenic
Cherries		Anti-angiogenic
Dark Chocolate		Anti-angiogenic
Magnolia Flower	Flos Magnolia	Anti-inflammatory
Lingzi Mushroom	Ganoderma Lucidum	Anti-inflammatory
Ginkgo Biloba	Ginkgo Biloba	Anti-angiogenic
Ginsing		Anti-angiogenic
Grapefruit		Anti-angiogenic
Green Tea		Anti-carcinogen
Kale		Anti-angiogenic
Red Sorrel	Hibiscus Sabdariffa	Anti-carcinogen
Lemons		Anti-angiogenic
Japanese Magnolia	Magnolia obovata	Anti-inflammatory
Chamomile tea	Matricaria Chamomilla	Anti-carcinogen
Holy Basil	Ocimum Sanctum	Anti-carcinogen
Licorice		Anti-angiogenic
Mitake Mushrooms		Anti-angiogenic
Nutmeg		Anti-angiogenic
Olive Oil		Anti-angiogenic
Omega-3 fatty acids		Anti-carcinogen
Oranges		Anti-angiogenic
Pineapple		Anti-angiogenic
Parsley		Anti-angiogenic
Pumpkin		Anti-angiogenic
Turmeric	Curcuma Longa	Anti-angiogenic
True Ginseng	Panax ginseng	Anti-inflammatory
Chinese Mushroom	Poria cocos	Immune System
Garlic		Anti-angiogenic
Grape Seed Oil	Proanthocyanidin	Anti-angiogenic
Onions and Fruit	Quercetin	Anti-inflammatory
Red Grapes		Anti-angiogenic
Resveratrol		Anti-angiogenic
Rosmary	Rosmarinus officinalis	Anti-inflammatory
Soy		Immune System
Strawberries		Anti-angiogenic
Tomatoes		Anti-angiogenic

Dr. Li's laboratory also tested the following four green teas:
1. Chinese Jasmine
2. Japanese
3. Earl Grey
4. A blend of Chinese Jasmine and Japanese

The Chinese Jasmine and Japanese teas by themselves were only half as potent as the Earl Grey. However in combination they had greater potency than the Earl Gray, which was twice as effective as either one of them by itself. This synergistic effect is often found in studies of anti-carcinogenic foods. Consuming a smaller quantity of many of the above food items every day would probably provide superior anti-angiogenic efficacy than concentrating on only one or two favorites.

What is remarkable about that list is that anyone who is into proper nutrition has already arrived at the same conclusion and has incorporated most of the above into their diets! It is however nice to have scientific proof. Petri dishes in the hands of ethical and unbiased bioresearch technicians seldom lie.

You can watch his lecture on angiogenesis at the following URL.

https://www.ted.com/talks/william_li

14 AMYGDALIN BASED CANCER TREATMENTS

In this chapter we will examine three of the most controversial cancer treatments. Normally they are considered to be three entirely different treatments for cancer but in reality all three of them are based to a great extent on amygdalin. The first thing we need to do is understand the difference between amygdalin and Laetrile. Amygdalin is a naturally occurring water soluble nitriloside the highest concentrations of which are found in apricot and bitter almond kernels. Laetrile is a highly concentrated extract of amygdalin which is injected into patients by alternative cancer clinics as a form of cancer treatment.

The consumption of apricot pits or bitter almonds requires no medical approval anymore than eating an apple would. Laetrile on the other hand is something quite different. It is a synthetically prepared and concentrated form of amygdalin usually administered through injection. There have been three studies performed on animals and two on humans that demonstrated some efficacy of amygdalin for the control of cancer but since there have been no universally accepted placebo-controlled and randomized clinical trials performed on humans Laetrile has not been approved by the FDA.

Although the preponderance of evidence indicates that the consumption of apricot kernels alone will not cure advanced cancer there is an enormous amount of anecdotal evidence which indicates that the daily consumption of a small quantity probably has a preventative effect. I personally know of several people who took 5-35 apricot kernels per day along with exercise as a part of their integrative treatment of cancer with excellent results. However the question still remains, how much of their cure was directly attributable to the consumption of amygdalin as opposed to the many other exercise and dietary elements that they included in their treatment.

There are tribal areas of West Pakistan were cancer does not exist. These people cultivate apricots for sale and consume large quantities of them themselves. The most prized part of the apricot in their culture is the kernel, which they always eat along with the apricot. this probably maintains a very high systemic level of amygdalin in their bodies which results in the absence of cancer within their population. Any native peoples that subsist to a large extent on wild rice, beans, berries and fruits show the same resistance to cancer. The Hunza tribes in Pakistan consume as much is 200 mg of amygdalin daily.

The cancer rate in the Philippines on the island of Mindanao were the diet consists mainly of cassava, wild rice and wild beans as well as a variety of berries and fruits is only one case per hundred thousand population. That is less than 1% of the US cancer rate. The Navajo and Modoc Indians of North America who routinely consume as much as 8 g of amygdalin per day are virtually cancer free. Cassava root can contain over 1,000 mg per kilo of amygdalin. Whenever any of these native peoples relocate and begin consuming our Western diet of sugar, white flour and other processed foods their cancer rate becomes equal to the Westerners with whom they are living.

In a study carried out by the Jyung Hee University in South Korea, amygdalin was reported to kill cancer cells in prostate cancer patients. The researchers declared it to be "a valuable option" in the treatment of prostate cancer (Biol Pharm Bull, 2006; 29: 1597–602).

In a separate study by a different team, but carried out at the same Korean university, amygdalin slowed the progress of colon cancer cells in test-tube genetic studies (World J Gastroenterol, 2005; 11: 5156–61).

Dosage: You should never consume more than six apricot kernels within 90 minutes. And a maximum of 35 per day. People with impaired liver function should be particularly careful with dosage. Today we do not consume barley, buckwheat and millet but instead have substituted refined wheat while pulses such as lentils from which we obtained 25% of our protein in 1900, now provide only 2%.

Here is a list of common plant sources of amygdalin

Alfalfa sprouts, Bamboo shoots, Mung bean sprouts

Barley, Buckwheat, Maize, Millet, Sorghum

Blackberries, Currants, Cassava, Cranberries, Loganberries, Yams Raspberries, Strawberries

Brown rice, Fava beans, Lentils, Kidney beans, Lima beans, Flaxseed and Linseed

Pecans, Macadamia nuts, Cashews, Walnuts, Almonds Watercress, Sweet potatoes

Lemon, Lime, Cherry, Apple, Apricot, Prune, Plum, Bitter almond and Pear seeds.

Animal studies:

In 1977 the SCIND Laboratories located in California conducted a study of amygdalin by dividing 40 cancerous rats into two groups of 20. One group was given three 200 mg injections of amygdalin, one every third day for a week. The mean survival time of the rats who received the injections was 70% greater than the control group. In another study that was conducted by Dr. Paul Reitnauer chief biochemists of the Manfred von Ardenne Institute in Dresden, Germany 20 out of a total of 40 mice were fed a diet that included bitter almonds which are high in amygdalin content. after 15 days of this diet all 40 mice were inoculated with 1 million abdominal cancer cells. the mice who had consumed a diet rich in amygdalin survived 26% longer than the control group.

In 1977, Dr. Vern L. van Breeman of Salisbury State College, Maryland conducted a study in which apricot kernels were feed to special strains of mice who were bred to develop breast cancer and leukemia. these mice lived 50% longer than the control group who did not received the amygdalin. While these studies do not prove that amygdalin is a cure for cancer they obviously show a very positive pattern of cancer growth suppression.

Human Studies:

Manuel Navarro, M.D., former professor of medicine and surgery at the Univ. of Santo Tomas in Manilla wrote in 1971: "I have specialized in oncology for the past eighteen years. For the same number of years I have been using Laetrile-amygdalin in the treatment of my cancer patients. During this eighteen year period I have treated a total of over five hundred patients with Laetrile-amygdalin by various routes of administration, including oral and I.V. The majority of my patients receiving Laetrile-amygdalin have been in a terminal state when treatment with this material commenced.

It is my carefully considered clinical judgment, as a practicing oncologist and researcher in this field, that I have obtained most significant and encouraging results with the use of Laetrile-amygdalin in the treatment of terminal cancer patients, and that these results are comparable or superior to the results I have obtained with the use of the more toxic standard cytotoxic agents."

In 1994, P.E. Binzel published his results from treating cancer patients with Laetrile. Between 1974 and 1991 He provided intravenous doses of 3 to 9 g of Laetrile to a group of 180 terminal cancer patients many of whom had been given up on by the Medical establishment and sent home to die. 138 of these patients were still alive in 1991 when he completed his study and published his results. Of the 42 patients who died only 23 had died from their cancers. The other deaths were from unrelated causes.

In October 2014 cancer researcher Jasmina Makarević showed that amygdalin dose-dependently reduced the proliferation of cancer cells in vitro.
http://journals.plos.org/plosone/article?id=10.1371/journal.pone.01 05590Jasmina Makarević

These are only a few of the testimonials by physicians and bioresearch facilities who have actually attempted to perform scientific studies into the efficacy of amygdalin and Laetrile. The fact that all of the studies have shown them to be effective in at least slowing down and inhibiting the progress of cancers even in stage IV patients is probably the reason why the mainstream medical establishment has resorted to terror tactics by claiming that people who take Laetrile or consume plants containing amygdalin are in danger of dying from cyanide poisoning.

All nitrileosides are three-part molecules consisting of sugar, cyanide and benzaldehyde. Although they contain an atom of cyanide it is no more dangerous than the chloride contained in table salt. normally the chlorine in Salt and the cyanide in Laetrile are both tightly bound and it is not possible for them to leak out and affect normal cells. The only thing within our bodies that can liberate the cyanide is the enzyme beta-glucosidase. Cancer cells contain 100 to 3,000 times more of this enzyme than healthy cells. When a molecule of amygdalin touches a cancer cell its' cyanide is liberated **killing the cancer cell.**

Cancer cells also contain a deficiency of rhodanese which detoxifies cyanide on contact producing thiocyanate. although rhodanese occurs throughout our bodies the majority of it is concentrated in our livers were most of the our blood detoxification occurs. Benzaldehyde also has anti-carcinogenic properties and has been used successfully by itself to treat various cancers providing up to a 50% reduction in tumor size. The combination of both benzaldehyde and cyanide are highly synergistic and have been proven to be effective against all types of cancer cells.

Is Laetrile safe?

Because cancer cells use anaerobic fermentation as a means of producing energy rather than the oxygen-based metabolism of normal cells they have a very different internal chemistry. Cancer cells have 3000 times the level of the enzyme glucosidase than that found in normal cells. This is the enzyme responsible for releasing the cyanide and benzaldehyde contained in amygdalin.

Healthy body cells contain the enzyme rhodenase, which when it encounters cyanide converts it into a harmless form called thiocyanate, which helps the body regulate both its blood pressure and vitamin B-12. This is why the small amount of cyanide that is released within our bodies from the breakdown of the amygdalin does not cause us any harm.

Research studies using adult mice have reported no health issues even at doses of 125 mg of amygdalin per day, Which is a high dose for a 170 lb. human let alone a mouse! They all lived to old age in perfect health none of them ever developing cancer. I guess in this case the "not developing cancer part" would be considered a "side effect" of the treatment. In 1981 Dr. Charles Moertal reported the results of a research study designed to prove how dangerous Laetrile is. However his report states:

"In our study, intravenous amygdalin was found to be free of clinical toxicity and no cyanide could be detected in the blood. In summation, the administration of amygdalin according to the dosages and schedules we employed seems to be free of significant side-effects. This conclusion appears to be validated by early observations in a phase II study of 44 Mayo Clinic patients receiving intravenous amygdalin therapy and 37 receiving oral therapy who have not experienced any symptomatic toxic reaction."

In an obvious display of their anti-laetrile bias Moertal concluded the summary abstract of their paper with the statement "A definite hazard of cyanide toxic reaction must be assumed." even though they state plainly in the conclusion of their report that they didn't find any Laetrile toxicity!

Be aware that no bitter almonds are currently allowed to be sold in the United States without first being pasteurized. This process renders the amygdalin completely ineffective. If the packaging claims they are raw they are telling the truth. The almonds have not been heated for a sufficient amount of time to cook them. They have only been super heated for a total of two seconds, which is just long enough to destroy the amygdalin content not cook them.

While amygdalin seems to be completely safe so far as cyanide poisoning is concerned be aware that byproducts of the cyanide process can build up in the liver. Usually cancer patient's livers are compromised in the first place and have very low levels of glucorinide which is the enzyme responsible for detoxification of the cyanide byproducts. For this reason the maximum dose of amygdalin should be limited to 1 gram. Even that small amount would probably consist of more apricot kernels than you would care to eat.

Conclusions:

Both naturally occurring amygdalin and Laetrile seem to have some efficacy in the process of curing cancers. However I do not believe that they are in and of themselves a reliable cure. Cancer patients become very proactive about doing everything they possibly can to become cancer free. This usually results in them using a shotgun approach and trying everything that could possibly help all at the same time. This is very logical and my own approach to curing my congestive heart failure was much the same and although it was extremely effective I really don't know what percentage of the overall recovery was due to the effects of which supplement. But in the end it is relatively irrelevant we simply need to keep using that shotgun method but at the same time make sure that the shotgun we use is as synergistic as possible.

Rene Caisse and Essiac

Rene M Caisse 1888-1978 was a Canadian nurse who treated cancer patients from the 1930s to the 1970s using a herbal recipe acquired from one of a local Indian tribes. This seems to be one of the most effective of all the alternative treatments with the most support of the medical establishment of the time. She successfully treated thousands of patients for end-stage cancers under the supervision of local physicians at no charge to the patients. The fact that she was providing this treatment free of charge and that she obviously believed in it herself proves that she was not a con artist and the fact that many physicians sent her their cancer patients to be cured indicates that the grassroots medical establishment believed in the efficacy of her treatment as well. The following is a narration by her chronicling the history of her treatment of patients.

"In the mid-twenties I was head nurse at the Sisters of Providence Hospital in a Northern Ontario town. One day one of my nurses was bathing an elderly lady patient. I noticed that one breast was a mass of scar tissue, and asked about it.

"I came out from England nearly 30 years ago" she told me. "I joined my husband who was prospecting in the wilds of Northern Ontario. My right breast became sore and swollen, and very painful. My husband brought me to Toronto, and the doctors told me I had advanced cancer and my breast must be removed at once. Before we left camp a very old Indian medicine man had told me I had cancer, but he could cure it. I decided I'd just as soon try his remedy as to have my breast removed. One of my friends had died from breast surgery. Besides, we had no money."

She and her husband returned to the mining camp, and the old Indian showed her certain herbs growing in the area, told her to make a tea from these herbs and to drink it every day. She was nearly 80 years old when I saw her and there had been no recurrence of cancer.

I was much interested and wrote down the names of the herbs she had used. I knew that doctors threw up their hands when cancer was discovered in a patient, it was just the same as a death sentence, just about. I decided that if I should ever develop cancer, I would use this herb tea. About a year later I was visiting an aged retired doctor whom I knew well. We were walking slowly about his garden when he took his cane and lifted a weed. "Nurse Caisse," he told me, "If people would use this weed there would be very little cancer in the world." He told me the name of the plant. It was one of the herbs my patient named as an ingredient of the Indian Medicine Man's tea!

A few months later I received word that my mother's only sister had been operated on in Brockville, Ontario. The doctors had found she had cancer of the stomach with a liver involvement, and gave her at the most six months to live. I hastened to her and talked to her doctor. He was Dr. R.O. Fisher of Toronto, whom I knew well because I had nursed patients for him many times. I told him about my herb tea and asked his permission to try it under his observation, since there was apparently nothing more medical science could do for my aunt. He consented quickly. I obtained the necessary herbs, with some difficulty, and made the tea. My aunt lived for 21 years after being given up by the medical profession. There was no recurrence of cancer.

Dr. Fisher was so impressed he asked me to use the treatment on some of his other hopeless cancer cases. Other doctors heard about me from Dr. Fisher and asked me to treat patients for them after everything medical science had to offer had failed. They too were impressed with the results. Several of these doctors asked me if I would be willing to use the treatment on an old man whose face was eaten away, and who was bleeding so badly the doctors said he could not live more than 10 days. "We will not expect a miracle," they told me. "Buy if your treatment can help this man in this stage of cancer, we will know you have discovered something the whole world needs desperately– a successful remedy for cancer."

My treatment stopped the bleeding in 24 hours. He lived for six months with very little discomfort. On the strength of what those doctors saw with their own eyes, eight of them signed a petition to the Department of National Health and Welfare at Ottawa, asking that I be given facilities to do independent research on my discovery. Their petition dated at Toronto on October 27, 1926, read as follows:

To Whom It May Concern: We the undersigned believe that the "Treatment for Cancer" given by Nurse R.M.Caisse can do no harm and that it relieves pain, will reduce the enlargement and will prolong life in hopeless cases. To the best of our knowledge, she has not been given a case to treat until everything in medical and surgical science has been tried without effect and even then she was able to show remarkable beneficial results on those cases at that late stage. We would be interested to see her given an opportunity to prove her work in a large way. To the best of our knowledge she has treated all cases free of any charge and has been carrying on this work over the period of the past two years. (Signed by the eight doctors)

I was joyful beyond words at this expression of confidence by such outstanding doctors regarding the benefits derived from my treatment. My joy was short-lived. Soon after receiving this petition, the Department of Health and Welfare sent two doctors from Ottawa to have me arrested for practicing medicine without a license. This was the beginning of nearly 50 years of persecution by those in authority, from the Government to the medical profession, that I endured in trying to help those afflicted with cancer. However, when these two doctors sent from Ottawa, found that I was working with nine of the most eminent physicians in Toronto, and was giving my treatment only at their request, and under their observation, they did not arrest me.

Dr.W.C.Arnold, one of the investigating doctors, became so interested in my treatment that he arranged to have me work on mice at the Christie Street Hospital Laboratories in Toronto, with Dr. Norich and Dr. Lockhead. I did so from 1928 through 1930. These mice were inoculated with Rous Sarcoma. I kept the mice alive 52 days, longer than anyone else had been able to do, and in later experiments with two other doctors, I kept the mice alive for 72 days with Essiac. This was not my first clinical experience. I had previously converted Mother's basement into a laboratory, where I worked with doctors who were interested in my treatment. We found that on mice inoculated with human carcinoma, the growth regressed until it was no longer invading living tissue after nine days of Essiac treatments.

This was during the period when I was working on DR. Fisher's suggestion that the treatment could be made effective if given by injection, rather than in liquid form, as a tea. I started eliminating one substance and then another. finally when the protein content was eliminated, I found that the ingredients which stopped the malignancy growth could be given by inter-muscular injection without causing the reaction that had followed my first experiments with injecting mice. However, I found that the ingredients removed from the injection formula, which reduced the growth of cancer, were necessary to the treatment. These apparently carried off destroyed tissue and infections thrown off by the malignancy. By giving the inter-muscular injection in the forearm, to destroy the mass of the malignant cells, and giving the medicine orally to purify the blood, I got quicker results than when the medicine was all given orally, which was my original treatments until Dr.Fisher suggested further experiments and developing an injection that could be given without reaction.

I well remember the first injection of the medication in a human patient. Dr. Fisher called and said he had a patient from Lyons, New York, who had cancer of the throat and tongue. He wanted me to inject ESSIAC ® into the tongue. Well, I was nearly scared to death. And there was a violent reaction. The patient developed a severe chill; his tongue swelled so badly the doctor had to press it down with a spatula to let him breathe. This lasted about twenty minutes. Then the swelling went down, the chill subsided, and the patient was all right,. The cancer stopped growing, the patient went home and lived quite comfortably for almost four years.

At the time I first used my treatment on terminal cancer cases or cancers that did not respond to approved treatment referred to me by the nine Toronto doctors I was still nursing 12 hours a day, the customary work day for nurses then. I had only my two-hour rest period and my evenings to give to my research work and my treatments. I decided to give up nursing to have more time for my research and treatment of patients. Doctors started sending patients to me at my apartment and I was treating about 30 every day.

I now felt I had some scientific evidence to present that would convince the medical profession my treatment had real merit. I made an appointment with Dr. Frederick Banting of the Banting Institute, Department of Medical Research, University of Toronto, world famous for his discovery of insulin. After reading my case notes, and examining pictures of the man with the face cancer before and after treatment, and x-rays of other cancers I had treated, he sat quietly for a few minutes staring into space. "Miss Caisse," he finally said, turning to look me straight in the eyes, "I will not say you have a cure for cancer. But you have more evidence of a beneficial treatment for cancer than anyone in the world."

He advised me to make application to the University of Toronto for facilities to do deeper research. He even offered to share his laboratory in the Banting Institute and to work with me. However, in making application to the University of Toronto, I would have to give them my formula, which could be filed in the archives and forgotten. Or could be used for university staff research and my application to do independent research at the university could still be refused

After much soul searching, I turned down Dr. Banting's suggestion and his offer to work with me. I wanted to establish my remedy, which I spelt Essiac (my name spelt backward), in actual practice and not in a laboratory only. I knew it had no bad side effects, so it could do no harm. I wanted to use it on patients in my own way. And when the time came, I wanted to share in the administration of my own discovery. To do such a thing is impossible even today for any independent research worker, due to what is nothing less than a conspiracy against finding a cure for cancer.

I decided to prove my treatment on it's own merit, without assistance if necessary. Dr. Banting approved my decision, and my courage. He had discovered insulin. He did not claim it was a cure for diabetes. He did know by experience that it was a palliative and a deterrent. I knew the same thing about ESSIAC ®. But Dr. Banting was a doctor and a recognized practitioner, so although he surrendered his formula to the profession under the medical code of ethics, he was honored and rewarded. I was in no professional position to secure acceptance of Essiac, or recognition for its discovery, if I surrendered the formula before the merit of the treatment was established beyond all doubt.

Tenants in my apartment house in Toronto objected to my numerous visitors the 30 or more daily patients. Besides I could no longer afford to carry on in the city any longer because I had given up nursing. I made no charge for my treatments and depended entirely on occasional voluntary contributions. I felt I could live less expensively in a smaller town, so I went to Timmins, thinking I would go back to nursing. However, Dr.J.A. McInnis(who signed the petition in 1926 and had seen my work in Toronto) asked me to treat cancer patients for him, which I did with good results.

I later moved to Peterborough, east of Toronto, and lived in a rented house, where I was no sooner moved in than the College of Physicians and Surgeons sent a health officer to issue a warrant for my arrest, again the charge was practicing medicine without a licence. I have lost count of the number of times I have been threatened with arrest and imprisonment for treating patients with Essiac. The health officer talked to me and some of my patients and then told me: "I am not going to issue this warrant, I am going back to talk to Dr. Noble, my chief". Dr. R.J.Noble was head of the College of Physicians and Surgeons.

The next day I wrote to the Hon. Dr. J.A. Faulkner, the Minister of Health, and asked for a hearing. I received a letter granting me a hearing on the following Monday at 2 p.m. I got in touch with doctors who had sent patients to me, and five of them together with 12 patients went with me to the hearing. We were received very graciously at Queens park by Dr. Faulkner, his deputy Minister The Hon. B.T. McGee and other doctors of National Health and Welfare.

After I presented my cases, Dr. Faulkner said that I could carry on, provided the patients came with their doctor's written diagnoses, and that I did not make a charge. My only ambition, I told Dr. Faulkner, is to prove Essiac on its merit, and make it acceptable to the medical profession."

So I started back for Peterborough, very proud and happy that I could continue to help patients. The look of gratitude I saw in their eyes when relief from pain was accomplished, and the hope and cheerfulness that returned when the saw their malignancies reduced, was pay enough for all my efforts. I had faith that if I trusted in God and did my best, a way to support my work would be found. I remembered our St. Joseph's Church in my home town of Bracebridge, Ontario, and the window in it dedicated to the memory of my mother, Fritzelda (Potvin) Caisse. She and my father raised their eight girls and three boys to love and fear God, and to believe that respect and love of our fellow man were more important than riches.

I never dreamed of the opposition and the persecution that would be my lot in trying to help suffering humanity with no thought of personal gain. I have never claimed that my treatment cures cancer– although many of my patients and the doctors with whom I have worked, claim it does. My goal has been control of cancer, and alleviation of pain. Diabetes, pernicious anemia and arthritis are not curable; but with insulin, liver extract and adrenal cortex extracts, incurables live out comfortable, controlled life spans. Cancer patients were successfully treated by me for over 25 years using ESSIAC hypodermically and orally. Since I am a nurse and not a physician, I never gave the treatment until I had a written diagnosis of cancer signed by a qualified doctor. I administered my treatment under the observations of doctors.

A few days after the hearing before the Department of Health and Welfare, Dr. Alfred Bastedo, of Bracebridge, called me. He had sent a patient to me with cancer of the bowel, and was greatly impressed with the results of my treatment. He told me he had gone before the Bracebridge Town Council and had asked that they offer me the old British Lion Hotel building to be used as a cancer clinic, if I would return to my home town to practice. He persuaded me to accept his offer. The Mayor and the Council of Bracebridge were very enthusiastic about getting the clinic started. With the help of friends, relatives and patients, I furnished an office, dispensary, reception room and five treatment rooms.

From 1934 to 1942, I paid the Council the sum of $1.00 per month for the building and there was a large "CANCER CLINIC" sign on the door. I treated thousands of patients who came from far and near, most of them given up as hopeless cases after everything in medical science had failed. Some arrived in ambulances, receiving their first treatments lying down in an ambulance; after a few treatments they walked into the clinic without help. I had absolute faith that I could accumulate enough proof of results obtained with different types of cancer, as demanded by the Cancer Society, the medical profession would eventually be glad to accept ESSIAC as an approved treatment.

I did not know then of an organized effort to keep a cancer cure from being discovered, especially by an independent researcher not affiliated with any organization supported by private or public funds. Tremendous sums have been raised and appropriated for official cancer research during the past 50 years, with almost nothing new or productive discovered. It would make these foundations look pretty sill, if an obscure nurse discovered an effective treatment for cancer!

About the time I opened my Cancer Clinic in Bracebridge, my own dear mother became ill. The four local doctors said she had gallstones, and her heart was too weak for surgery. Mother was 72 years old at the time. As she got worse, I insisted on calling Dr. Roscoe Graham, a consulting specialist of international fame, for an examination and consultation with the other doctors. After the consultation, Dr.Graham came to me and said: "Your mother has cancer , Miss Caisse. Her liver is a nodular mass." Dr.McGibbon, local doctor who was set against my cancer work, said very sarcastically, "Why don't you do something?" I'm certainly going to try, doctor, I replied. I asked Dr.Graham, How long does she have to live? Dr.Graham thought it would only be a matter of days.

I immediately started treating her with Essiac. I gave it daily for 10 days. When she improved I reduced the treatment to three a week, then to two, then to one. She continued to improve. To make a long story short, my mother completely recovered. She passed away quietly after her 90th. Birthday– without pain, just a tired heart. This repaid me for all my work giving my mother 18 years of life she would not have had without Essiac. It made up for the great deal of persecution I have endured at the hands of the medical world.

A few doctors in the United States became sufficiently interested in ESSIAC to investigate the treatment. Some people from Chicago who knew my work persuaded DR. John Wolfer of the Alumni Association of Northwestern University at Chicago, to have me treat patients in a Chicago clinic under the observation of their doctors. A consultant specialist took me to see Dr. Wolfer and read the histories of the cases selected for my treatment all hopeless or terminal. I looked the histories over and asked "when would you like me to start, doctor?" He looked surprised because, as he told me later, he had expected me to turn them down.

I arranged to be in Chicago to treat these patients each Thursday, under supervision of five doctors. The consulting specialist asked me, as he took me back to the home of friends in Chicago, why I had accepted these terrible cases "I will show results that will surprise your doctors, even in these late stages of the disease." I told him. "The results will be enough to interest even the most skeptical doctors." I was proved right. Later, these doctors offered to open a clinic for me in the Passervant Hospital in Chicago, if I would stay in the United States.

Dr.Richard Leonardo, a surgeon specialist and coroner of Rochester, N.Y., at first scoffed at the idea of any merit in my work. "The only way to prove or disprove the merit of Essiac," I told him, "Is to remain in the clinic and see the patients and observe my work and the results." He decided to do so. The first day he stayed and talked to patients; then he told me he was satisfied that I was getting results, but it was my faith and encouragement that brought hope and improvement to my patients not my treatment. "These results are entirely psychological" he stated emphatically.

The second day I invited him to come into my treatment room, examine patients and watch me administer the treatment. We had many advanced cases of cancer and I did not finish in the clinic until 7:30 pm. He stayed until the last patient left. "Young lady," he told me, "I must congratulate you. You have made a wonderful discovery." Dr.Leonardo stayed for four days examining patients and becoming more and more interested in my results. "I like your method of treatment," he said. "I feel it will change the whole theory of cancer treatment and will eventually do away with surgery, radium and x-ray treatments for cancer." He offered to establish and equip a hospital in Rochester if I cared to move there and work with him.

Both of these offers to establish clinics in the United States were tempting, but my forebears on both sides of my family had come to Canada from France in the 1700's and I had made up my mind long ago that Canada would get the credit for providing a cure for the world's most dreaded disease. Dr.Leonardo's investigation of my treatment was during the summer of 1937, while Dr. Emma H.Carson of Los Angeles was spending June and July of that year visiting my Bracebridge Clinic and studying the treatment and it's result.

The following report is by Dr. Emma Carson of Los Angeles, CA., dated August 12, 1937:

Several of my world-renowned professional friends (physicains, surgeons and attorneys) and also four famous business officials were spending the winter of 1936-37 in Southern California, and upon various occasions when they visited me I learned of Miss Caisse's wonderful cancer clinic at Bracebridge, Ontario. Owing to such glowing and impressive reports and the intense interest so earnestly evidenced during these discussions, I became interested. I then expressed a resolve to go to Bracebridge as soon as introductory letters could be exchanged, providing Miss Caisse would invite me to visit her clinic. The invitation was most cordially extended including explicit instructions for my convenience and comfort, her genuine assurance of sincere welcome and her appreciation of the fact that I was coming from a great distance to investigate her work, regardless of my sceptical attitude.

At 8a.m. on the fourth day after receiving her welcome invitation, I left Los Angeles, en route to Bracebridge for the exclusive purpose of meeting Miss Rene M. Caisse and ascertaining the real virtue of her Essiac treatments, according to her invitation, and especially appreciative of her promise to demonstrate her method and system personally in her clinical work. As I seriously and compassionately surveyed that extraordinary assembly of afflicted people and visually compared them with the most prominent and distinguished clinics I have ever witnessed either in this or foreign countries, I vividly realized I had never before seen or been in any way associated with such a remarkably cheerful and sympathetic clinic, regardless of size, location or number of persons; or attended a more peaceful, sympathetic clinic anywhere.

I was also assured by patients that they voluntarily abandoned narcotics and sedatives of every denomination, that had been prescribed to them by their physicians who had attended them previous to their adoption of Essiac treatments, and very soon after the first treatment of Essiac. My skepticism neither yielded nor became subdued by the hopes and faith so definitely expressed by the Clinic patients and their friends. However, I candidly admit that my curiosity became greatly augmented, and I resolved that skepticism should not blind my eyes or oppose my thorough investigation of the real efficacy of the Essiac treatment for cancer.

Several prominent physicians and surgeons, who are quite familiar with the indisputable results obtained in response to Miss Rene M. Caisse's Essiac treatments, and who have also asserted their great interest in cancer research work, including the investigation of the most prominent advocated remedial treatments for cancer, really conceded to me that Rene M. Caisse's treatment is the most humane, satisfactory and frequently successful in consideration of her unavoidable limitations due to certain restrictions remedy for annihilation of cancer that could be found at that time. I candidly explained the motive that determined my visit to the Bracebridge Cancer Clinic. I hoped to obtain visibly authenticated proof that would sufficiently convince and satisfactorily establish incontrovertible evidence of Essiac as a reliable remedial agent for cancer.

Miss Caisse explained her earnest desire to conscientiously provide all verified information, both favourable and unfavourable, to aid and establish unbiased and impartial conclusions, decisively confirmed, as a merited compensation for my long distance trip, made for the purpose of obtaining convincing evidence concerning the real merits of Essiac. I diligently proceeded in quest of the definitely assured results accomplished by the use of Essiac, and attributed to miss Rene Caisse's treatment for cancer. I firmly resolved that my investigation must be based on unprejudiced judgement.

Miss Caisse does not even suggest "cure all" pertaining to her Essiac remedy. When asked if Essiac will cure cancer, she always replies: "If it does not cure cancer it will afford relief, if the patient has sufficient vitality remaining to enable him to respond to treatment." The vast majority of Miss Caisse's patients were brought for treatment after surgery, radium, emplastrums, etc. had failed to be helpful and the patients pronounced incurable or hopeless cases. Really, the progress obtainable and the actual results from Essiac treatments and the rapidity of repair were absolutely marvelous, and must be seen to convincingly confirm belief.

I was intently engaged in reviewing, comparing and summarizing my accumulation of data, records, histories, etc. and mentally visualized each patient and his apparently miraculous progress toward recovery, when I realized that skepticism had deserted me, or in recognition of defeat folded its tent, like the Arabs, and silently passed away. When I arrived in Bracebridge, I contemplated remaining 12 hours, at least not more than 48 hours. Miss Caisse and her Essiac treatment and her patients were responsible for the unlimited extension of my time in Bracebridge and Toronto, as I remained 24 days and spent about 16 days at Toronto. During the three weeks of the time I visited Bracebridge and neighbouring cities and towns, I investigated and examined results obtained by Essiac treatments including 400 patients.

I am pleased to assure all interested parties that I paid my own expenses and investigated Essiac to satisfy my own interest in cancer victims and learn of some remedial agent for cancer that had proved itself superior in every respect to all else, and which I could conscientiously recommend to my friends and interested persons. I can certainly express my genuine regrets that Ontario is so far away and difficult to reach for cancer sufferers from California. Transportation covering such long distances is certainly an important consideration for the safety and comfort of invalids. With sincere interest and hopes that humanity throughout all nations be permitted to obtain Miss Rene Caisse's remedy ESSIAC according to her philanthropic and humane principles, I remain,

(Signed : Emma M.Carson, M.D., Hayward Hotel, Los Angeles, California, August 12, 1937)

Every few years I would make an appointment with whoever was then The Honourable Minister of Health for Ontario and would attend with a group of patients and a petition. First Dr.Robb, then Dr. Faulkner and the Honourable Harold Kirby. Each year the group of patients would be more numerous, and the petitions would carry more names. The last petition was presented in 1938 with a bill requesting our government to legalize my Essiac treatment. This bill was presented to the 2nd. Session of the 20th. Legislature of Ontario, 1938, for "An act to authorize Rene Caisse to practice medicine in the Province of Ontario in the treatment of cancer and conditions resulting therefrom." The Bill was sponsored by two members of the provincial legislature from opposing political parties Mr. J.Frank Kelly, a member of the Liberal Party and Mr. Leopold McCauley, a member of the Conservative Party. There were 59 voting members in the legislature and the bill failed by only three votes. It would have authorized the practice of the treatment of cancer without a medical rating. This was a position never before heard of in the history of Canada.

I learned later that this unusual bill, authorizing me to practice medicine in the treatment of cancer, would, no doubt, have actually been approved by the Legislature, except that members of the medical profession assured the members that if the bill was not passed they would not sponsor the appointment of a Cancer Commission to give my treatments a fair hearing. It came to light later that the Canadian Medical Association had debated my case with the legislature before my hearing and had made this false promise. Soon after the hearing of my bill, the Legislature passed "An Act For The Investigation Of Remedies For Cancer" This act established the Cancer Commission and among other things, provided that:

"The Commission may require any person, who advertised, offers for sale, holds out, distributes, sells or advertises either free of charge or for gain, hire or hope of reward, any substance or method of treatment as a remedy for cancer, to submit samples of such substance or a description of such treatment, and samples of such substance used with such treatment to the Commission together with the formula of such substance and such other information pertaining to such substance or method of treatment as the Commission may determine" I immediately closed my clinic, and reopened it only at the urgent request of the Minister of Health, The Honourable Harold J.Kirby and the Premier of Ontario, The Honourable Mitchell Hepburn.

The Honourable Mitchell Hepburn said at the time this bill was passed: "The onus is on the medical profession now. They must either prove or disprove Miss Caisse's claims, and I do not believe they can disprove them. I am in sympathy with Miss Caisse's work and will do all in my power to help her"

The Premier answered an inquiry from Mrs. Wilfred Raney, of Sunbridge, Ohio about my treatment, stating that I could carry on as in the past. From the Office of the Prime Minister of Ontario and dated June 8, 1938, it read: Dear Mrs Raney: In reply to your letter of recent date relative to miss Rene Caisse's cancer cure, I wish to advise you that the Commission for the investigation of so-called cancer cures has not been set up as yet. Miss Caisse is in the same position today as she was prior to the passing of an Act for the Investigation of the Remedies for Cancer. There has been no interference whatever by the department of health, nor by any department of the government. The Minister of Health and the deputy Minister have personally interviewed Miss Caisse, and she has been advised that she can carry on her treatment in the meantime the same as she has done in the past. With kind regards, I remain Yours very sincerely (Signed Mitchell Hepburn)

Eventually on December 31, 1939, the Commission into the Investigation of Cancer Remedies brought in its report which read in part, "After careful examination of all the evidence submitted and analysed herewith and, not forgetting the fact that the patients , or a number of them, who came before the Commission, felt they had been benefited by the treatment which they had received, the Commission is of the opinion that the evidence adduced does not justify any favorable conclusion as to the merits of Essiac as a remedy for cancer and would so report."

It is my opinion, that the hearing of my case before the Commission was one of the greatest farces ever perpetrated in the history of medicine. More than 380 patients came to be heard, and the Commission limited the hearings to 49 patients. Then, in their report stated that I had only 49 patients to be heard! They stated that x-ray reports were not acceptable for diagnosis, and that the 49 doctors had made wrong or mistaken diagnosis. It is a sad state of affairs if doctors can diagnose an affliction as cancer and send the patients home with a few months (at most) to live, if they are not sure. In the 49 cases examined by the Commission, the majority had been diagnosed by more than one physician. Some of them had three or four doctors, and were told they had cancer, and were treated for malignancy before coming to me for Essiac treatment.

In the hearing, the Cancer Commission admitted that every patient presented had benefited or been cured by Essiac, many of them with pathological findings and reports, but they said the doctors had been mistaken in diagnosing the cases. More than 300 patients were waiting to be heard but the Commission stated they had seen enough to give a report. The Cancer Commission made much of the fact that I had not furnished them with the formula of Essiac or with samples thereof. What they did not state was that I had been offering to the proper authorities for years my formula providing they would admit some merit for Essiac on the clinical proof I presented. I had offered to give it to them if they assured me that it would not be shelved (as was done with penicillin). So I did not give out my formula and they published the bald statement that "I refused to give my formula."

My files reflect hundreds of documented cases concerning the proven efficacy of Essiac with cancer patients, including many of the 49 that the Cancer Commission turned down for dubious reasons. I will give just two cases of patients who appeared the Commission in July of 1939, and who were alive and well 20 or more years later.

Patient 1. Walter Hampson, Utterson, Ontario, aged 34 in 1937. Diagnosis: squamous carcinoma of lip. Physicians; Dr. Ansley, Pathologist, and Dr. A.F. Bastedo, Bracebridge, Ontario.

After the pathologists report, Dr. Bastedo urged Mr. Hampson to go at once to have radium treatment as he had no time to lose. Mr. Hampson came to me for treatment and was cured. When he went before the Cancer Commission on July 4, 1939, with other patients, they listed his case as "Recovery due to surgery." The only surgery he had was the removal of a small section for the biopsy which showed the cancer! Mr. Hampson was well on May 4, 1960.

Patient 2. Herbert Rawson, Bracebridge, Ontario. Age 48 in 1935. Diagnosis: carcinoma of rectum, confirmed by x-ray.

Patient had a hard mass with sloughing and bleeding and great pain. When he refused surgery, Dr. Kenny gave Miss Rene Caisse a written diagnosis with permission to treat with Essiac. Treatments began in April of 1935 and the last of 30 treatments was given on May 1, 1936, and a good improvement in weight. Patient was able to work during treatment period except for one month of rest. No trace of cancer was found in 1936 when he was examined by doctors W.C. Arnold of Ottawa, Herbert Monthorne of Timmins, Ontario and F.Greig of Bracebridge, Ontario. May 22, 1960, Mr. Rawson , 73, died of a stroke.   In 1963, Mrs. Carline Donald, 79, and John McNee,95, died. Both had been cured of cancer at the Bracebridge Clinic, but no doubt the investigators would now claim that they never did have cancer. It seems the only cases they admit had cancer are the ones who died of it, in spite of all the research and conventional treatments.

The Prime Ministers, The Ministers of Health and later the Cancer Commissioners and the Attorneys-General of Ontario received hundreds of letters and pleas from patients and their doctors regarding Essiac. Many of the 55,000 persons who signed the petition supporting the bill to recognize and legalize my treatment, also wrote letters. The Cancer Commissioners, backed by certain medical groups, were deaf to the appeals, and used the same biased interpretations of data as have been placed on other treatments indicated for cancer, unless limited to their approved surgery, radiation and toxic drugs."

Renée returned to her hometown and continued treating patients on a personal basis until her death in 1978.

How to make Essiac Tea

The following recipe is from Mali Klein's website (www.essiacfacts.com). It is an excellent source of information on all aspects of using Essiac for the treatment and prevention of cancer. She lists a couple of sources for Essiac powder on her site that are very reasonably priced. Another very good website is:

(http://www.theoriginalessiac.com). They also sell Essiac in its' final liquid form ready to drink.

The recipe for Essiac tea.
1-1/2 tablespoons (80 grams) of powdered Sheep Sorrel (Rumex Acetosella)
2 tablespoons (120 grams) of finely chopped Burdock Root (Arctium Root)
2 teaspoons (20 grams) of powdered Slippery Elm inner bark. (Ulmus Vulva)
1/4 teaspoon (5 grams) of powdered Indian Rhubarb (Rheum Palmatum)

All of the ingredients should be certified organic. The sheep sorrel is the most important and all of it should be used (leaves, stems and roots). Only the root of the burdock plant is used and if you are going to grind your own make sure that it is fresh because once it dries out it is too difficult to cut or grind. You should purchase the Slippery Elm bark already ground. The Indian Rhubarb is easy to grind. Freshness of the ingredients does not seem to be an issue so purchasing all of them dried and pre-ground should not reduce the potency.

Cardinal Rules for preparation and storage

Always store both the powder and the finished tea in a refrigerator in a tightly sealed jar.

Always sterilize all utensils by boiling for 20 minutes prior to use.

Always make sure the lids are on the bottles before you put them in the refrigerator.

Never leave open bottles out of the refrigerator.

Microwaving or freezing will destroy the tea's potency. Microwaving has been proven to alter the molecular structure of any type of nutrient or food that is exposed to it.

Preparation of the ingredients

First wash and dry your hands carefully after removing any rings from your fingers. Make sure that whatever you use to dry your hands is fresh and bacteria free as well.

Place the 5 grams of turkey rhubarb root into a dry clean bowl and add the 20 grams of slippery elm bark powder. Use your fingers to blend these two ingredients together very well so that they stick to each other. This will make sure that the small amount of rhubarb root is evenly distributed throughout the finished powder.

Add the 80 grams of sheep sorrel powder mixing everything together with your fingers again. Followed by the 120 grams of burdock root continuing to mix all four ingredients together with your fingers for even distribution. Place the resulting powder in a quart mason jar and store in the refrigerator.

To prepare a batch of tea from the powder you will need a stainless steel pot (never use aluminum or Teflon coated) that will hold 3 quarts of water without boiling over. Do not use this pot for any other purpose save it solely for making your tea.

Use 15 grams of herb mixture to 1 1/2 liters of water. This is enough to provide one person 1 ounce (30 grams) per day for a month. You cannot use tap water as there are too many toxins in it. It is best to use is a natural mineral water that has a very high pH around of around seven. This will also help to keep your systemic body pH alkaline. If that option is not available then steam distilled water would be the next best choice.

Pour one and a half liters of water into your pan and add the 15 g of herb mixture thoroughly stirring it into the water. Bring to a boil and reduce the flame to a very low rolling boil for 10 minutes.

While you're waiting for the mixture to boil use a bottle brush to thoroughly clean out three one pint (500ml) brown glass bottles that you will store the tea in as well as the stainless steel sieve that you will be using to strain the mixture. These items should only be used for your tea preparation as well.

After 10 minutes turnoff the flame and scrape off any of the powder residue that has stuck to the sides of the pot and stir it into the solution. Cover the pot with its' lid and allow the solution to steep for 10-15 hours but not longer than 18 hours.

Before pouring the liquid into its half liter bottles you will need to sterilize all of the implements you will be using by boiling them for 20 minutes. This is absolutely necessary because the tea contains no preservatives and will be stored in your refrigerator for as long as a month giving bacteria and other organisms the opportunity of growing in the mixture if it is not completely sterile. never use bleach or any other chemicals to do the sterilization as their residue will be transferred to the Tea.

Now we need to reheat the tea in the pot so that it just starts to steam. Never bring it to a boil of any kind as that will weaken the effect of the solution. As soon as it starts to steam remove it from the heat and let it sit until all of the herbs have settled to the bottom of the pot. then use a strainer to strain the liquid into your sterilized measuring cup and then pour it into your sterilized brown glass storage bottles.

Never filter the tea, only strain it through a standard stainless steel mesh kitchen strainer to keep from removing too much of the particulate matter contained in the liquid. Place your three brown glass bottles of tea in your refrigerator for daily use throughout the rest of the month. If after 5 - 7 days you notice a fur-ball growing on the sediment in the bottom of the bottle it means that you failed to sterilize everything properly and the only solution for this problem is to pour it down the drain and have another go at doing it correctly.

You prepare the solution for drinking by placing one fluid ounce (30 ml) into a cup or glass and then adding 2 fluid ounces (60 ml) of hot but not boiling water. The tea should be a light yellow to medium brown but never a dark brown color. Sometimes the burdock root will turn it a bright green color depending upon its source, this is not a problem.

The dosage is once per day preferably prior to bedtime and can be consumed on a full or empty stomach. It is really quite pleasant and does not taste bitter. Don't forget that if your pet has cancer you can provide them with about a 45 ml dose per day by placing the tea in their water dish and hopefully it will help cure them as well.

Harry Hoxsey

Harry Hoxsey was an ex-coal miner with only an eighth grade education. He was the recipient of an herbal remedy for cancer that had been passed down through his family from his great-grandfather, which proved to be very effective. His great-grandfather was a veterinarian whose prize stallion came down with cancer so he put it out to pasture and waited for it to die. In three weeks however the tumor stabilized and then begin to recede.

He made observations of which plants the horse ate and discovered that it was grazing on plants that it normally would not eat if it was well. So he compounded a formula to treat his animal patients and had very good results with it. He passed this treatment down through his family until it arrived at Harry.

By the 1950s the Hoxsey Clinic in Texas was the largest cancer treatment facility in the world with subsidiaries in 17 states. This eventually attracted the interest of the FDA as well as the local authorities who threatened him with legal action. This turned into one of the longest running legal battles in the history of alternative medicine. Not only was Hoxsey a very stubborn Texan but unlike Rene Caisse also had acquired sufficient wealth through his oil and ranch businesses that he could afford the legal expenses required to keep the government hounds at bay.

Hoxsey was able to afford to compile credible data such as x-rays and pathological studies to prove that his treatment worked. He also had a well established network of local doctors, senators, judges and politicians who endorsed his treatment. Hoxsey was arrested more than 100 times in Texas by Attorney General Al Templeton. But when Templeton's own brother came down with cancer and was cured by Hoxsey Templeton was converted from enemy to friend and became his lawyer. Juries in two separate federal trials acquitted him of medical fraud on the basis of finding overwhelming evidence that his methods were both safe and highly effective cures for cancer.

During the trials none of his more than 10,000 patients were willing to testify against him.

Hoxsey offered to have the AMA come to his facility and conduct whatever research tests that they needed to convince themselves that his procedures were effective. The AMA refused to examine the Hoxsey cure, or evaluate it for either safety or efficacy because they were afraid that it would legitimize his work. They simply stated that they knew from their own education in medicine that the treatment he was offering was completely ineffective so they didn't need to test it.

At the same time that the medical authorities were trying to shut him down members of the AMA were offering to purchase Hoxsey's formula for a large amount of money. Hoxsey refused for the same reason Renée Caisse did, the AMA would not guarantee that it would be made available to anyone who needed it free of charge if they could not pay.

After that the AMA attacked Hoxsey relentlessly for the next 20 years trying to prevent him from curing people of cancer. Rather than trying to settle the dispute by scientific testing they instead used their control of the medical media and newspapers to slander Hoxsey and his cure. Hoxsey by this time had brought in so many oil wells that he could afford to fight back. He eventually sued Dr. Fishbein head of the AMA for slander. Although it was thought to be impossible for Hoxsey to win his lawsuit, he eventually did and Fishbein was forced to resign from his post at the AMA. Fishbein eventually admitted that Hoxsey's treatment did in fact cure cancers.

Ultimately the FDA padlocked the doors of all seventeen of his clinics shutting them down and he did not have sufficient funds to fight all seventeen of the cases at the same time. He finally established a clinic in Mexico which continued to treat thousands of patients and is still active today. Their patients have to go across the border into Mexico to receive their medications and are only allowed to bring enough of it back to the United States with them for their own use.

Ironically, Hoxsey's own treatment failed to cure his own cancer. He eventually turned to chemotherapy and died within seven years of liver toxicity from the chemotherapy drugs. In one last parting insult from the medical establishment, his death was recorded to have been from cancer. These foods are avoided when on the Hoxsey therapy: tomatoes, vinegar, pork, alcohol, table salt, sugar, and white flour.

The ingredients for his cancer treatment consisted of:

Wild Indigo Root (Babtisia Tinctoria)

Red Clover Blossom (Trifolium Pretense)

Licorice Root (Glycyrrhiza Glabra)

Buckthorn Bark (Rhamnus Cathartica)

Burdock Root (Arctium Lappa)

Stillingia Root (Stillingia Sylvatica)

Poke Root (Phytolacca Americana)

Barberry Root Bark (Berberis Vulgaris

Oregon Grape Root (Berberis Aquifolium)

Cascara Sagrada Bark (Rhamnus Purshiana)

Prickly Ash Bark (Xanthoxylum Americanum)

Kelp (Laminaria Species) or Bladderwrack (Fucus Vesiculosus)

Potasium Iodine was supplemented separately as well.

The hoxsey treatment is still being provided by the clinic he set up in Mexico. Their website is (http://www.hoxseybiomedical.com).

Conclusions

If you were given to experimentation as a child you probably tasted several different types of wild grasses and weeds. They are almost universally bitter. This is because nearly all of them contain high levels of the amygdalin. This is why I placed Hoxsey's and Caisse's treatments in this chapter. They both utilize wild grasses, barks and herbs that contain amygdalin.

This is probably the main effective ingredient in their formulas for the treatment of cancer. If you are not currently symptomatic for cancer simply remembering to eat the seeds of any fruit you consume, especially apricots and peaches, as well as apples will provide you with additional protection against cancer. If you already have cancer then acquiring large quantities of unpasteurized apricot kernels and consuming larger doses would be a good idea. The essiac tea is relatively easy to prepare and could be combined with green tea as a cancer preventative as well.

Neither Rene Caisse nor Harry Hoxsey ever turned away patients because they were poor. Their service was provided free to cancer patients who could not afford to pay.

15 DIETARY CANCER TREATMENTS

If poor diet can cause cancer, perhaps a healthy one can cure it.

As we've already read in an earlier chapter the ellagiac acid contained in most berries is a powerful anti-angiogenic substance as well as being an antioxidant. Most cancer patients If they decide to change their diet at all will use faulty information acquired either from friends and family or the tabloids rather than performing legitimate research into the topic and selecting a diet that is very low in carcinogens and high in anti-carcinogens. Usually this will involve going vegetarian because they've heard that meat is carcinogenic despite the fact that there is no research proving that this alone will increase their chances of survival.

Conventional wisdom quite often is very compelling to the point of being very difficult to refute unless you want to take the time to go on pubmed, learn Latin and read the legitimate medical research papers that are peer-reviewed and tend to tell the truth. The sad fact is that the majority of people who develop any form of major illness are suffering from malnutrition.

Women with breast cancer inevitably have low blood plasma levels of vitamin C and B12 as well as omega-3 fatty acids and minerals such as magnesium, selenium, potassium and calcium. Along with this they usually have low oxygenation of the blood plasma due to lack of exercise along with very high salt and sugar intake which produce high systemic acid levels.

One of the most contentious of all the diet oriented cancer cures is the Gerson therapy. The popular press tends to attack this form of alternative cancer treatment by asking ignorant questions such as "How could coffee enemas or large doses of vitamin C cure cancer?" In reality the Gerson therapy makes no such claims about either. Both are simply a small part of their overall treatment strategy which revolves around the systemic purging of toxins within our bodies and especially within our livers thereby returning our physical health to the natural balance that nature intended it to have. Charlotte Gerson has recently modified the Gerson therapy so that it incorporates the findings of the latest cancer research.

Then there is Dr. González of New York whose therapy consists of 120 different supplements each of which is administered to correct some nutritional imbalance in your body chemistry. His primary interest is focused on pancreatic enzymes. He has conducted his own clinical trials and achieved excellent results from his therapies. The problem with all of these alternative cancer treatments is that there has been very little or no mainstream research into their efficacy. Without sufficient unbiased research studies none of these alternative treatments will ever be accepted by oncologists.

The real problem is that there is so much infighting amongst the various factions whether they are representing their own particular alternative cancer treatment or being attacked by mainstream media as quackery. What we desperately need are some adults on all sides of the issue who can sit down and maturely discuss the real science involved without bringing their political or economic views into the discussion. This infighting benefits no one least of all the cancer patients. The treatment of cancer is a multistep multifaceted process and the end result is too important to trust solely to one dogma.

Ellagic Acid

Ellagic acid is a relatively new type of cancer therapy that uses concentrated ellagic acid derived from red berries and pomegranates. In one in-vitro study, it dose dependently killed pancreatic cancer cells at levels of between 180 - 900 mg/dl and slowed cancer cell growth by 20 times at the higher dosage.
(World J Gastroenterol, 2008; 14: 3672–80).

In another study using mice, pomegranate-derived ellagic acid stopped the growth of prostate cancer cells. (J Agric Food Chem, 2007; 55: 7732–7)

Anthocyanins: These are found in blueberries, cherries, cranberries and red currants as well as vegetables such as red cabbage and beetroot

Ellagic acid: It is found in grapes, pomegranates, raspberries and strawberries. This is an antioxidant, which moderates the effects of estrogen. This is especially important for men.

Lycopene: Tomatoes are the main source of lycopene. It is one of the strongest antioxidants and is particularly effective against colorectal cancer. Unlike many other anticancer nutrients tomatoes must be cooked in order to release their lycopene.

Pterostilbene: Found in blueberries and grapes. It is similar to resveratrol and likewise is highly protective against genetic damage to our DNA.

Resveratrol: Found in red grapes, blueberries and pomegranates. not only does it help to prevent cancers but is one of the most potent anti-aging nutrients available at a reasonable price. To gain the maximum benefits per dose you must open the capsule and empty the powder into the space between your gum and lower lip so that it can be completely absorbed directly into the bloodstream. This will result in a systemic blood level two hundred times greater than if you had swallowed the 1 g capsule. It takes about three months to see the results which are really quite impressive judging by my own experiences.

The ORAC rating system

Scientists have developed a rating system for comparing the amount of protection from oxidative stress that various fruits and vegetables provide. It is the ORAC score. ORAC stands for Oxygen Radical Absorbance Capacity. The right-hand side of the table below shows the ORAC rating for various types of berries. The scores for various vegetables on the right-hand side of the table show that berries are in general a more concentrated source of antioxidants than vegetables.

Berry	ORAC Rating
Goji Berries	25300
Kale	1770
Cranberries	1750
Broccoli	890
Strawberries	1540
Beetroot	841
Raspberries	1220
Red Pepper	713
Plums	949
Onion	450
Cherries	670
Cauliflower	377
Acai Berry	18500
Spinach	1260
Prunes	5770
Brussels Sprouts	980
Blueberries	2400

Alfalfa Sprouts	930
Blackberries	2036

One of the most enjoyable ways to incorporate a variety of these beneficial fruits into your diet is to go to one of the websites that features recipes for fruit smoothies and start blending.

The Gerson cancer treatment

The Gerson dietary cure for cancer was developed by Dr. Max Gerson (1881-1959). During his early 20s he suffered from severe migraine headaches and began experimenting with dietary changes to see what effect they would have on his condition. He soon discovered that a salt free vegetarian diet kept him free of his migraines. After he graduated from medical school and became a physician he would recommend the same diet to patients who came to him with migraines. Eventually one of his patients reported that not only were his migraines cured but his skin tuberculosis as well.

Skin tuberculosis was untreatable at that time so Dr. Gerson started treating skin tuberculosis patients for free using his diet with very good results. He was then invited to try his cure at a tuberculosis Institute in Munich Germany which resulted in the cure of 445 out of 450 patients. A few years later he cured Albert Schweitzer's wife of lung tuberculosis using the same treatment. Over the next few years his studies indicated that not only was his diet curing the targeted disease but also most all of the more minor ailments that these patients had such as high blood pressure, allergies, asthma and kidney problems. When he tried to use his diet to treat cancer he soon discovered that the rate of efficacy was only about 40%.

Further research indicated that there was a difference between patients suffering from general chronic diseases and those who had cancer. Those that suffer from chronic diseases had damaged livers whereas those who suffered from cancer had toxic livers which need to be restored to health prior to starting the nutritional therapy.

When Schweitzer was 75 years old he developed diabetes and was cured by Gerson's treatments as well. The treatment is one that cleanses the entire body through the use of organically grown vegetable and fruit juices while avoiding all types of meat Once cleansed the human body is then able to cure itself of what every ailment may be present including cancer.

Max Gerson eventually had to leave Germany and move to New York to escape persecution by the Nazis. On July 1-3 in 1946 he testified before the Senate. The evidence presented by him and his patients was so compelling that the most famous radio announcer in New York Raymond Gram Swing announced to the entire United States that finally a cure for cancer had been discovered. The public response was overwhelming.

Two weeks later Swing was fired from his position of 30 years as a radio announcer at ABC. He was a victim of the AMA. One of the reasons that the AMA hated Gerson was that he was the first physician to denounce cigarette smoking as a cause of cancer. Unfortunately the cigarette company Philip Morris was one of the main advertising contributors to the AMA journal. He was ostracized from the entire medical community.

Over the next 10 years he wrote a book that documented 50 cases of terminal cancer that had been sent home to die that he had cured. The reason that established medicine was so vehemently opposed to his treatment was that it was nutritional therefore not profitable but at the same time highly successful which would've put them out of business. He finally retired to an apartment in New York and continued to cure cancer patients on an individual basis until his death.

Estimates by various physicians suggests that the death rate from cancer in the United States would be cut in half if his therapy were allowed to be performed here. The Gerson Clinic is now located in Mexico and has a continual flow of cancer patients from all over the world who receive treatment and recover as a result of it. The medical records of more than 1500 patients are available to anyone that cares to examine them.

According to the Gerson clinic their treatment is most effective against the more aggressive forms of cancer such as melanoma, ovarian and lung cancer. The reason for this may be that because these more aggressive cancer cells physically deviate the most from normal cells it is easier for the patients newly recovered immune systems to recognize and kill them. One of the primary tenants of the Gerson therapy is a continuation of the diet even after the malignancy has disappeared. The theory is that if the patient has allowed his immune system to become so dysfunctional that cancer occurred in the first place then an extended period of time is necessary for complete recovery and then a lifetime maintenance regime to maintain their immune system health. If you are interested in trying this approach Charlotte Gerson's book "Healing the Gerson Way" is available on Amazon.

Approved Foods: Un-sulphureted dry fruits, oatmeal, Garlic, vinegar, lemon juice.

Regulated Foods: Less than 2 teaspoons of sugar per day in the form of honey, maple Syrup or molasses.

Disapproved foods: Spices, Berries, Soy, Tofu

Procedures: Coffee enemas

It is interesting that spices and berries which have been proven to control cancer are prohibited.

16 INTEGRATIVE APPROACH

Many research studies have proven that our lifestyles can impact our genetics almost as much as the original genetics that we inherit from our parents. In 2009 researchers at the University of Montréal studied a group of women whose genetics predispose them to an 80% chance of breast cancer during their lifetimes. They determined that women who carry this gene but consume a wide variety of fruits and vegetables every week had a 75% lower chance than the control group of having breast cancer.

This and other studies seem to indicate that cancer producing genes contained within our chromosomes are not nearly as dangerous if they are not triggered by an unhealthy lifestyle. Additional studies in this area have indicated that women who lived prior to 1945 had three times less risk of developing breast cancer than their granddaughters who live in the fast food culture of today. Apparently the so-called cancer genes are simply genes that have a poor tolerance for improper nutrition.

Dr. Dean Ornish has become famous for his studies in the area of integrative cancer treatment. In 2005 he published the results of a study he conducted on 93 men who had prostate cancer that had been confirmed by biopsy. These men had decided not to undergo surgery or other treatment of their cancers. Dr. Ornish decided to use them to study the efficacy of natural integrative treatments for their cancers. He divided the patient's into two groups. The control group would simply be observed by their physicians and receive PSA tests to determine the progress of their cancers.

Over the course of the one-year study the second group would receive vitamins E and C as well as selenium. They also received 1000 mg of omega-3 fatty acids daily. In addition to the supplements they exercised by walking 30 minutes per day and practiced stress management. For the majority of these cancer patients this was a major lifestyle change. Most of the parameters being studied were considered by oncologists to be irrational and irresponsible.

At the end of the study the 49 patients in the control group who had simply continued their lives as usual showed a 6% increase in their PSA levels where as the patients in the second group who had been proactive about changing their lifestyles averaged a 4% decrease in their PSA levels indicating a regression of their prostate cancers. Six of the control group patients ultimately required surgery, chemotherapy and radiation to control their cancers while the members of the second group did not require any further conventional treatments.

But what was even more impressive was the fact that blood drawn from members of the second group was seven times more capable of inhibiting the growth of prostate cancer cells en-vitro. The final critical piece of information concerning the study is that the more diligent the patients in the second group were about following the lifestyle change guidelines the more affective their blood was at inhibiting the growth of cancer cells.

Dr. Ornish then initiated an additional study to determine what genetic changes had occurred within the RNA of the patient's who had undergone lifestyle change. The end results of this study which was published in 2008 indicated that his lifestyle change program had modified the actual function of more than 500 genes in the prostate gland. It stimulated prostate genes which inhibited cancer growth. As it turns out diet and lifestyle changes can have a profound effect upon our genetics. This by the way is called the science of epigenetics.

Although no natural approach to curing cancer can be considered 100% effective the bottom line is that unlike conventional treatments such as chemotherapy the natural approaches are 100% healthy and beneficial to the body and its defenses so even if a patient decides to resort to chemo, radiation or surgery there is no logical reason why he should not embrace the natural approaches as well. The detoxification of our bodies of known carcinogenic substances and the consumption of foods that have proven to be anti-carcinogenic should be a no-brainer for anyone. In addition to curing cancer the implementation of many of these dietary, emotional and mental changes will greatly increase the quality and quantity of our lives regardless of whether we suffer from cancer or not.

Whether or not cancer will occur depends greatly upon the existence of cancer promoters and anti-promoters. Even if there is an abundance of promoting agents within our genetics this can be more than offset by the existence and/or reinforcement of anti-promotion agents. Epigenetics also plays a very important role in whether or not cancer becomes expressed within an organism or not. Cancers are very much like weeds in a garden. If the type of soil is conducive to the growth of weeds they will tend to prevail and it is only when we change the basic composition of the soil that the good plants that we are trying to grow will start to prevail over the weeds.

Most of these cancer promoters are provided by our diets. They are those agents that promote systemic inflammation such as insulin and IGF-I. In the same manner our diets can provide us with anti-promoters which greatly reduce the odds of our bodies ever allowing a cancer to get out of control and become dangerous. Quite often plants contain agents which protect them against the perdition of insects and fungus. Likewise various agents such as green tea, coffee, berries and tomatoes are highly protective against cancer.

Green tea in particular contains a molecule called epigallocatechin gallate (EGCG). It has been determined that this particular molecule is extremely anti-angiogenic. EGCG provides a protective coating for cells which makes it very difficult for pathogens to attack and penetrate our cell membranes. It also prevents the new formation of blood vessels which a cancer would normally use to feed itself and grow. Three or 4 cups of green tea per day is an excellent anti-carcinogenic. Green teas also aid in the detoxification of our livers. The two most beneficial things that we can do for our livers is to drink relatively large quantities of both green tea and coffee and utilize coffee enemas to detoxify them.

Our livers need to deal with the elimination of the many environmental toxins that find their way into our bodies either through direct contact with our skin, inhalation or being inadvertently consumed in our foods. Tests have shown that the possibility of a prostate cancer growing to an advanced stage are reduced by 50% when men consume at least 5 cups of green tea per day. This is one of the more pleasant ways to prevent cancer. Olives contain numerous antioxidants which assist in the prevention of cancer and this could well be why the Mediterranean diet is so effective in both cancer prevention and heart health.

One of the best natural anti-inflammatory foods is turmeric. This is the primary ingredient in yellow curry in both Indian and Thai cuisine. Laboratory research has indicated that it inhibits the growth of a large variety of cancer cells. It is also highly anti-angiogenic and promotes cancer cell apoptosis. Consuming turmeric by itself in capsule form unfortunately is not affective. Consumption of pepper as well as ginger at the same time is required to enable it to be absorbed through the intestinal wall. Curries are fairly simple to cook so perhaps that would be a more enjoyable way to consume turmeric rather than swallowing a pill. When this meal is accompanied with green tea the anti-cancer effects are very synergistic.

Japanese shiitake, maitake, enokitake and kawaratake, mushrooms contain polysaccharides which stimulate the immune system.

17 OTHER ALTERNATIVE TREATMENTS

The Johanna Budwig Protocol

Dr. Johanna Budwig (1908-2003) was a well-respected biochemist and physicist as well as an expert on the pathology of cancer. During her research into the metabolism of fats and oils within our bodies she determined that hydrogenated, trans and even polyunsaturated fats could cause fatty deposits in the coronary arteries blocking circulation to the heart. They also inhibited cell membrane renewal and disrupted the normal flow of liquids through the lymphatic system.

One of her main areas of research was on the increased levels of cancer due to insufficient levels of essential lipoproteins and phosphatides in the modern Western diet. Her own research and that of her fellow scientists proved that the consumption of flaxseed oil in and of itself would compensate for the deficiencies of the modern diet. During the course of these studies she found that it could even cure certain types of cancer.

Her research indicated that the blood of terminal cancer patients was a greenish-blue rather than a red, indicating a lack of hemoglobin oxygenation. Nobel Prize winner Otto Warburg won his Nobel Prize in 1931 for demonstrating the importance of proper oxygenation in preventing cancer. His research demonstrated that cancer cells could not survive in the presence of oxygen.

Dr. Budwig found that several months of daily treatment with flaxseed oil altered her patients' blood chemistry sufficiently through the increased presence of lipoproteins and phosphatides that a decrease in tumor size resulted. She ultimately determined that beneficial fatty acids such as Omega-3 needed to freely pass through cell membranes if they were to be utilized by those cells. In order to do this she bound the beneficial lipids to sulfur in order to make them water-soluble. The simple mechanism she arrived at for accomplishing this was to mix the ground up flaxseed with cottage cheese so that the oils contained in it would bind to the sulfur bearing proteins of the cottage cheese thereby allowing them to pass through the cell membranes uninhibited.

As is so often the case with alternative cancer treatment practitioners her patients tended to be those who had already been treated with the orthodox chemotherapy and radiation and were in the final stages of cancer metastasis some of which had only days left to live. There are literally thousands of testimonials from people around the world who were diagnosed with terminal cancer and then completely cured by her simple cottage cheese and flaxseed treatment.

Research studies both in the United States and Japan have shown that women whose urine contains the highest levels of flaxseed also have the lowest levels of breast cancer. Secoisolariciresinol is the natural lignin found in flaxseed which attenuates the metabolism of estrogen and the ability of estrogen to bind to its receptors throughout the body. Secoisolariciresinol prevents estrogen from accelerating the growth of cancer cells. It also causes an increase of "Sex hormone binding globulin", which also reduces the amount of free estrogen that is available to stimulate cancer cell division.

Two research studies using animals given a cancer-inducing chemical demonstrated that 46% fewer as well as smaller tumors occurred in the group that also received Secoisolariciresinol. Tests on women with breast cancer showed that factors associated with tumor growth fell 35 per cent in the group whose diet included flaxseed.

The Budwig Recipe

Put 5 tablespoons of ground flaxseeds or flaxseed oil in a blender along with 1 cup of organic, low fat cottage cheese. Fruit can be added especially strawberries. Blend the mixture for a couple of minutes and let it set for about 15 minutes before consuming.

Mistletoe

Mistletoe (Iscador) is an herbal remedy purported to have cancer-fighting qualities, according to Rudolf Steiner's school of anthroposophical medicine and is usually given as an injection. However, because of the controversy surrounding its' use in the US. research has been confined to a few cancer centers in Europe.

Three new studies suggest that it can be very helpful in slowing the growth of cancer cells, as was predicted by Steiner. In a set of four clinical trials, Iscador-treated patients with ovarian cancer survived longer than the control group regardless of whether the cancer had spread. (Arzneim Forsch, 2007; 57: 665–78).

Iscador demonstrated similar anti-carcinogenic effects in patients with cervical cancer (Forsch Komplement- XXXrmed, 2007; 14: 140–7).

Finally, in a case report of a 68-year-old man with malignant melanoma that had spread to his liver was successfully treated with Iscador from 1999 until he was completely cured in 2002 with no recurrence since then (J Altern Complement Med, 2007; 13: 443–5). (Arzneim Forsch, 2007; 57: 665–78).

Ozone therapy

Ever since Dr. Warburg discovered that cancer cells can only exist in the absence of oxygen considerable research has been done trying to figure out different ways to increase the oxygenation of a cancer patient's body. I suppose that simply doing daily exercise is just too difficult a concept to implement so they need to complicate it as much as possible. Ozone therapy has actually been a mainstream medical treatment for many years in Germany. Ozone is an unstable molecule consisting of three atoms of oxygen. As well as being one of the most powerful oxidizers it is also a disinfectant and antibiotic which is often used for sterilization of room atmospheres.

Used properly it is highly beneficial for patients with serious illnesses because it increases their blood oxygen levels at the same time killing many pathogens especially in the lungs. It is of course illegal to use in the United States despite its having been proven to be completely safe and to increase the cure rate for cancer in European studies. This is an especially beneficial treatment for patients of any kind who have impaired uptake of oxygen or who are living at higher altitudes where there is less oxygen per breath. The following abstract is from a research paper published June 10 2015 on pubmed.gov. At the bottom of the abstract is the resource locator if you want to read the entire research paper.

Abstract
"The Warburg effect and tumor hypoxia underlie a unique cancer metabolic phenotype characterized by glucose dependency and aerobic fermentation. We previously showed that two non-toxic metabolic therapies the ketogenic diet with concurrent hyperbaric oxygen (KD+HBOT) and dietary ketone supplementation could increase survival time in the VM-M3 mouse model of metastatic cancer. We hypothesized that combining these therapies could provide an even greater therapeutic benefit in this model. Mice

receiving the combination therapy demonstrated a marked reduction in tumor growth rate and metastatic spread, and lived twice as long as control animals. To further understand the effects of these metabolic therapies, we characterized the effects of high glucose (control), low glucose (LG), ketone supplementation (βHB), hyperbaric oxygen (HBOT), or combination therapy (LG+βHB+HBOT) on VM-M3 cells. Individually and combined, these metabolic therapies significantly decreased VM-M3 cell proliferation and viability. HBOT, alone or in combination with LG and βHB, increased ROS production in VM-M3 cells. This study strongly supports further investigation into this metabolic therapy as a potential non-toxic treatment for late-stage metastatic cancers."

http://www.ncbi.nlm.nih.gov/pubmed/26061868

Skin Cancer Cure

I have used this to eliminate three Basal Cell Carcinomas, which account for 80% of all cancers. They all healed perfectly with no scaring and there have been no recurrences as of one year later. This procedure is simple to implement and from my experience 100% effective for treating basal cell carcinomas as well as actinic keratosis and squamous cell carcinomas. The basic rule of cancer eradication is "If you can touch it you can kill it." Cancer cells are extremely fragile and can be killed by applications of substances that are actually beneficial to the surrounding normal skin cells.

1. Buy some ascorbic acid powder. This is the most effective substance to use. It will kill the cancer cells and be beneficial for the surrounding non-cancerous skin cells as well. It is very selective and when applied as an aqueous paste will capillary down into the cancer roots and kill them as well but spare the surrounding normal cells.

2. Wet about one level teaspoon of ascorbic acid with water to form a paste. This should be enough for the entire treatment. Do not use

anything but water for the wetting agent. Some use coconut oil which will not capillary down into the cancer roots and kill them. Skin is 75% water, coconut oil and water do not mix.

3. Apply the paste to the BCC.

4. Place a cloth type Band-Aid over the BCC to keep the paste from coming off. Moisten the Band-Aid at regular intervals to keep the ascorbic acid paste under it from drying out.

5. Continue until the BCC is gone and the skin is scabbed over.

6. This should take about 4-6 days.

7. Discontinue the ascorbic acid application and remove the band aid.

8. Wait for the scab to come off in a week or two.

Many studies have demonstrated that topical anti-carcinogens including ellagic acid and olive oil (polyphenols) are effective against skin cancer as well.

Anti-neoplaston therapy

This treatment was pioneered by Dr Stanislaw Burzynski, a Polish physician and scientist who is now practicing in Houston, Texas. The treatment is based on the observation that cancer patients are deficient in certain amino-acid compounds called peptides. Burzynski has discovered a technology for manufacturing peptides, which are then injected into cancer patients with the belief that these peptides will cause cancer cells to revert to healthy ones. In one study, 74% of children with low-grade gliomas (brain tumours) saw a marked improvement in their condition, while 91%of patients with colon cancer who were given the therapy were still alive after five years compared with just 39 per cent of those who had received the usual chemotherapy (Integr Cancer Ther, 2004; 3: 47–58).

In a case report of a 40-year-old man with a brain tumor, whose prognosis was very poor, anti-neoplastons were administered for 655 consecutive days. As of four years after the end of treatment, the patient is still completely cancer free. (Integr Cancer Ther, 2004; 3: 257–61).

I almost didn't include this particular treatment because to me it reeks of snake-oil salesman. There are however at least two research papers which seem to indicate that it is effective. The other thing that made me finally decide to include it is that the US Government after granting him permission to do clinical trials with this preparation then proceeded to persecute this poor man for nearly 30 years for doing it!

As far as I'm concerned anytime the US government goes after any kind of alternative treatment with that kind of enthusiasm the treatment is probably credible. Also after trying to revoke his medical license for the last 15 years the state of Texas finally has given up and allowed him to treat patients. At this point he is one of the few if not the only alternative cancer treatment physician who has tacit permission to practice in the US.

18 CANCER PROOFING YOUR LIFESTYLE

"It really is true that you can't see the forest for the trees."

Many of you will be disappointed in this final chapter believing that I should have provided more details about how to fine tune your lifestyle to prevent cancer. If I did that I would be guilty of over complicating a very simple subject. The problem is that because of the seeming inability of the worlds most brilliant research biologists to find a solution most people think that curing cancer is a very complex problem. This is only true if you are trying to find a chemical based cure for cancer.

All of the pharmaceutical laboratories are currently working on chemical versions of the natural cures listed in this book. They know they work they are just trying to find an active ingredient who's molecular structure can be altered just enough so that it will be patentable. At this point you should have a very good understanding of what causes cancer as well as the numerous options for preventing it. The only thing left for us to do is figure out practical ways to incorporate what we have learned into our personal health programs.

There are three basic aspects of anticancer nutrition. The first is the consumption of foods and nutrients that support immune system health. The second, which is equally important is the consumption of foods and nutrients that have proven to be anti-carcinogenic. The third is the avoidance of carcinogens both in the foods we consume and our environment.

Behaviors to eliminate

1. Stop drinking carbonated beverages, period!

1. The carbonation greatly increases the body's systemic level of acid.
2. The sugar in them will create systemic inflammation.
3. If it is artificially sweetened the sweetener is a carcinogen.

There is no upside to drinking carbonated beverages.

2. Stop using sugar in any form!

It is the worst thing you can do to your body short of eating rat poison. The inflammation that it causes is systemic. Most cases of arthritis and rheumatism as well as many other diseases that have inflammation as their main symptom are caused by this. The only exception to this rule is the small amount of fructose that naturally occurs in the fruit you eat. Do not try to substitute refined fructose for sucrose as it is even more inflammatory than sucrose. If you buy the refined version and try to use it like table sugar it will do the same damage to your body as sucrose.

3. Eliminate as many high glycemic foods as possible.

After about a month when your metabolism has adjusted to the elimination of carbonated beverages and sugar begin eliminating the remaining high glycemic foods from your diet as much as possible. At the same time gradually increase your consumption of fat and low glycemic vegetables so that your body can gradually switch over to utilizing fat for energy instead of carbohydrates.

Removing those three things from your life will reduce your chance of becoming a cancer victim by at least 50% not to mention curing just about every other inflammatory problem you have such as arthritis.

4. Eliminate as many carcinogens from your life as possible.

5. Stop consuming processed foods and learn to cook.

6. Reduce the amount of time you spend talking on your cellphone and message more.

7. Because of the large amounts of mercury, radiation and chemicals that they have absorbed the consumption of large game fish such as tuna and swordfish is probably not a good idea. Substitute freshwater fish instead.

8. Avoid consumption of monosodium glutamate.

9. Only use meat products that do not contain nitrites or nitrates.

10. Avoid any GMO produce and food products obtained from animals that were fed GMOs.

11. Avoid all high glycemic index foods such as white rice, wheat and potatoes that will spike insulin levels. Use brown rice, whole wheat and sweet potatoes instead.

12. Eliminate as much body fat as possible.

13. Minimize your exposure to x-radiation.

14. Eliminate stress from your life as much as possible.

15. Check the ingredient labels on all of your household products for xenoestrogens. See page 78 for list.

16. Don't rush in to conventional treatments such as chemotherapy no matter how much pressure the oncologist places on you. As we have seen, studies have proven that it can take as long as two years for our immune systems to finally get around to dealing with a cancer and that the survival rate for people who decide not to do chemotherapy is at least twice as long as the people that undergo chemo. Spontaneous regression of cancers happens far more often

than people realize and should not be eliminated as a possibility as long as the cancer patient maintains his immune system at an optimum level of efficiency.

17. Limit your consumption of meat to ten ounces per week.

Behaviors to implement

1. Regular daily exercise combined with 4 cups of green tea or coffee per day. In a study that used four groups of mice it was shown that caffeine induces cancer cell apoptosis and that this effect is synergistic with exercise. The first group of mice received no caffeine or exercise. The second group received caffeine but no exercise and had a 100% increase in cancer cell apoptosis over the first group.

The third group received exercise but no caffeine and had a 120% increase in cancer cell apoptosis over the control group. The fourth group received both exercise and caffeine and had a 400% increase in cancer cell apoptosis. Coffee served with a generous helping of exercise is one of the most beneficial things that you can do for your body.

2. Maintain the proper levels of magnesium, calcium and potassium. The best way to supplement potassium is by taking a potassium iodine tablet every few days, which will help maintain your thyroid health as well. If you're using a potassium sparing diuretic the potassium you receive from foods will probably be sufficient.

3. Learn to prepare Thai or Indian foods. so that you will receive the anti-carcinogenic benefits of both the spices and the coconut oils used in their preparation.

4. Eat moderate quantities of berries throughout the week as well as other fruits that provide anti-angiogenic and anti-inflammatory protection.

5. Be certain that all of your eggs, fish and meat products are free range and organic so that you have a better chance of maintaining a proper Omega-6 to Omega-3 ratio of at least 4 to 1 (ideal is about 2 to 1).

6. Substitute olive and coconut oils for vegetable oils when cooking as well as butter for margarine.

7. Try to buy most of your produce from organic sources as it does make a tremendous difference.

8. Preform monthly checks of your body PH to make sure that it is 7.5 or higher.

9. Daily consumption of amygdalin containing seeds from apples apricots and bitter almonds as well as an ounce or two of Essiac Tea.

10. Incorporate Dr. Johanna Budwig's cottage cheese and flaxseed cancer preventative into your diet. Adding the berries that you plan on eating that day will act as a flavor enhancer.

11. All that is required to incorporate parts of the Gerson diet therapy into your anticancer regime is a juicer and enema equipment. Juicing helps break down vegetable and fruit cellular walls and release the nutrients contained inside them.

12. If you have any clothing dry cleaned you should be sure to allow them to air out for several hours prior to wearing to avoid contact absorption of the chemicals through your skin.

13. Every time we prepare a meal we have very critical choices to make. We can select foods that promote cancer cell apoptosis and help prevent angiogenesis within cancer cell clusters preventing metastases or we can continue to consume foods that support the development of cancers.

14. Eating foods that are anti-inflammatory will reduce the ability of cancer cells to inflame the surrounding healthy cells and trick our

bodies into thinking that there's an injury in that area that requires the generation of new capillaries to feed the new tissue which in this case happens to be malignant. We also need to consume foods that provide the nutrients that detoxify our bodies of carcinogenic substances. Anti-carcinogenic foods are fully capable of overcoming any toxic carcinogens that we take in but we first need to consume them in sufficient quantities that they are able to provide that function for us.

Ketogenic fat loss

The remainder of this book is dedicated to people who have always wanted to lose fat but have been unable to achieve that goal. This is a distillation of my current experimentation in maintaining a 10% or lower body fat percentage. It really isn't difficult and is one of the most important things that you can do to reduce your risk of becoming a cancer victim. It will also help prevent heart disease.

Our bodies were designed for life, as it was 100,000 or more years ago. Agriculture had not yet been invented so there was no continuous supply of calories available to keep us going. We were hunter-gatherers who might have a surplus of food one day and none for the next four. To cope with this our bodies developed the ability to store energy in the form of fat and then utilize that stored energy for fuel when no food was available.

Carbohydrates in whatever form are first used to make blood glucose. When our bodies have enough to supply our current energy needs, the remainder is turned into fat for future use. There are only two types of sugar that can cross the brain blood barrier and nourish it, glucose and ketones. After about 14 hours without carbohydrates our blood glucose levels become low enough that our bodies switch over to converting our fat stores to ketones.

Obviously blood glucose depletion happened on a regular basis when we were hunter-gatherers. This was not normally a problem since our bodies would simply switch over to converting fat to ketones, which were then used for energy until we were able to find a source of carbohydrates and once again increase our blood glucose to high levels. If we were lucky we would have enough left over to store some as fat for later use.

A good analogy is an automobile's gas tank. When we fill it up we are limited to the capacity of the tank. Normally we do not keep trying to put gas in if it is running back out the filler pipe onto the ground. We then drive the car using the gasoline stored in it's tank until such time as the tank is close to empty when we fill it again and repeat the cycle.

It is the same with our bodies, our fat cells are our gas tank and we convert the fat contained in them to ketones as we look for more carbohydrates to replenish our fat stores so that they can provide energy in the future when we can't locate a food source. Unfortunately our bodies have a limitless gas tank. They simply add more fat cells to contain any extra blood glucose that is produced from the carbohydrates that we consume. Our fat cells are the perennial pessimists of our bodies and are always preparing for the next famine.

Until recently our systemic levels of glucose have always been very low. Because carbohydrates and pure sugars were so difficult to find our diets consisted mainly of proteins and fats, which supplied our immediate energy needs very well but could not be stored for future use. Sugars were in the form of fruit, which was often out of season and honey, which was very painful to collect. To compensate for this our bodies developed an insatiable craving for anything sweet because it could be easily converted directly into fat so that we would have reserves of energy to fall back on during the lean times.

Fast forward to the modern era. We use fewer calories to maintain our bodies because of our easier workloads but at the same time we have readily available sources of cheap high glycemic food to store as fat. This makes our bodies very happy because they have an endless supply of carbohydrates to convert into fat for the future famine, which never occurs. The processed food industry uses our natural obsession with carbohydrates as a marketing tool to sell us their products by incorporating sweetness into them.

We have so lost touch with reality that we think that being in ketosis is a bad thing that can be solved by simply eating something. In reality having low blood glucose and using our fat stores for energy is historically our normal state and not something to be avoided.

The Ketogenic Diet

Ketogenic diets are very effective for fat lose and many of the recipes are delicious as well as easy to make. Because of the richness and caloric density of Ketogenic foods you will eat less often and consume a smaller quantity at each meal. When in ketosis 50-70% of our calories should come from good fats such as the medium chain triglycerides found in coconut oil and avocados.

Once your body has adjusted to obtaining its energy from fats instead of glucose start reducing the amount of food you consume and your body will switch over to the consumption of your body fat to replace that caloric deficit.

Once you are in ketosis stay there by not eat more than 50mg of carbs per day, the equivalent of 2 slices of whole wheat bread. I view the hard core Ketogenic diet as temporary. It can be used to loose large quantities of fat quickly, after which you can switch to a more varied one such as the Mediterranean diet, which has been proven to reduce fatal heart attacks by 70%.

Here are some lists of common Ketogenic foods

Proteins	Calories	Fats g	Net Carbs g	Protein g
Bacon, 1 oz	176	14	0	12
Steak, 1 oz	69	4	0	7.7
Beef, 1 oz	70	4.3	0	7.2
Chicken, white, 1 oz	49	1.3	0	8.8
Chicken, dark, 1 oz	58	2.8	0	7.8
Egg, 1 oz	46	3	0.25	4
Fish, 1 oz	20	0.1	0	4.3
Fish, Salmon, 1 oz	40	1.8	0	5.6
Ham, 1 oz	50	2.6	0	6.4
Hot dog, 1 oz	92	8.5	0.5	3.1
Lamb chop, 1 oz	39	0	7.3	6.0
Pork chop, 1 oz	65	4.1	0	6.7
Pork ribs, 1 oz	102	8.3	0	6.2
Scallops, 1 oz	31	0.2	1.5	5.8
Shrimp, 1 oz	28	0.1	0	6.8
Tuna, 1 oz	52	1.8	0	8.5
Turkey Breast, 1 oz	39	0.6	0	8.4
Veal, 1 oz	42	1	0	8

Vegetables	Calories	Fats g	Net Carbs g	Protein g
Asparagus 1 oz	6	0.1	0.6	0.7
Avocado, 1 oz	47	4.4	0.6	0.6
Broccoli, 1 oz	10	0.1	1.1	0.7
Carrots, 1 oz	10	0	1.5	0.01
Cauliflower, 1 oz	7	0.1	0.5	0.5
Celery, 1 oz	5	0	0.3	0.7
Cucumber, 1 oz	4	0	1	0.2
Garlic, 1 clove	4	0	1	0.2
Green beans, 1 oz	10	0.1	1.3	0.5
Mushrooms, 1 oz	6	0.2	0.6	0.9
Onion, white, 1 oz	11	0	2.1	0.3
Bell Pepper, 1 oz	6	0	0.8	0.2
Pickles, dill, 1 oz	3	0	0.4	0.2
lettuce, 1 oz	5	0.1	0.3	0.4
Shallots, 1 oz	20	0	3.9	0.7

Peas, 1 oz	24	0	2.8	1.5
Spinach, 1 oz	7	0.1	0.4	0.8
Squash, Acorn, 1 oz	16	0	2.9	0.3
Squash, 1 oz	11	0	2.1	0.3
Tomato, 1 oz	5	0	0.8	0.3

Diary Product	Calories	Fats g	Net Carbs g	Protein g
Buttermilk, 1 oz	18	0.9	1.4	0.9
Cheese, Blue, 1 oz	100	8.2	0.7	6.1
Cheese, Brie, 1 oz	95	7.9	0.1	5.9
Cheese, Cheddar, 1 oz	114	9.4	0.4	7.1
Cheese, Colby, 1 oz	110	9	0.7	6.7
Cheese, Cottage, 1 oz	24	0.7	1	3.3
Cheese, Cream, 1 oz	97	9.7	1.1	1.7
Cheese, Feta, 1 oz	75	6	1.2	4
Cheese, Monterey	106	8.6	0.2	7
Cheese, Mozzarella, 1	85	6.3	0.6	6.3
Cheese, Parmesan, 1	111	7.3	0.9	10.1
Cheese, Swiss, 1 oz	108	7.9	1.5	7.6
Cheese, Marscapone, 1	130	13	1	1
Cream, half-n-half, 1	39	3.5	1.3	0.9
Cream, heavy, 1 oz	103	11	0.8	0.6
Cream, Sour, 1 oz	55	5.6	0.8	0.6
Milk, whole, 1 oz	19	1	1.5	1

Nuts and Seeds	Calories	Fats g	Net Carbs g	Protein g
Almonds, 1 oz	170	15	3	6
Brazil Nuts, 1 oz	186	19	1	4
Cashews, 1 oz	160	13	7	5
Chestnuts, 1 oz	55	0	13	0
Chia Seeds, 1 oz	131	10	0	7
Coconut, 1 oz	65	6	2	1
Flax Seeds, 1 oz	131	10	0	7
Hazelnuts, 1 oz	176	17	2	4
Madadamia Nuts, 1 oz	203	21	2	2

Peanuts, 1 oz	157	13	37	0
Pecans, 1 oz	190	20	1	3
Pine Nuts, 1 oz	189	20	3	4
Pistachios, 1 oz	158	13	56	0
Pumpkin Seeds, 1 oz	159	14	1	8
Sesame Seeds, 1 oz	160	14	4	5
Sunflower Seeds, 1 oz	150	11	4	3
Walnuts, 1 oz	185	18	2	4

Intermittent Fasting

Intermittent fasting is a great tool for loosing fat and is very synergistic when combined with the Ketogenic diet. You eat dinner a couple of hours before going to bed. If you eat at 8:00 pm and go to bed at 10:00 pm for example you would probably wake at around 6:00 am. At this point you have been fasting for 10 hours and your goal is to not consume anything but water until around 2:00 am in the afternoon. This is not as difficult as it seems. You can add green tea to the water along with stevia and a squeeze of lemon. If you can only make it to noon the first couple of days that is fine, just keep trying to extend the length of your fast by thirty minutes each day.

When you are finally able to make it to 2:00 you will have fasted for 18 hours and you can then eat enough Ketogenic food to just satisfy your immediate hunger so that you can make it to 8:00 pm for your next Ketogenic dinner just prior to bedtime. Combining a Ketogenic diet with intermittent fasting is one of the quickest and most effective means of loosing fat, especially if you are getting regular exercise as well. The website www.leangains.com is the place to go for information on this type of program.

Fat Cell Apoptosis

If you follow the advice about Ketogenic dieting and intermittent fasting you will probably find that you initially lose a very large volume of fat but that when you have lost about two thirds of the fat you started out with you suddenly stopped losing the remaining 30%. There is a very simple and logical reason for this. At this point you have very little fat stored in the remaining fat cells. They are empty but like empty one liter water bottles the cells themselves still take up space. It is only possible to lose two thirds of your fat volume by dieting alone.

At this point you need to remain on your no carb diet and wait until your body decides that you no longer will need those empty fat cells for future fat storage. The problem is that our bodies are programed to expend as little energy as possible and preemptively destroying all of those billions of fat cells would require our bodies to expend a great deal of energy. The end result is that our bodies take a wait and see approach and allow the fat cells to die of old age rather than taking an active role in eliminating them. Since all of the cells in our bodies are replaced every 3 to 5 years that much time will have to pass before all of them are eliminated.

This does not mean that you will carry the remaining empty fat cells and the bulge around your waist that they create for five more years at which point they will all disappear overnight. Some have already reached the end of their useful life span and will immediately begin to die so it will probably take about 2 years to lose most of that remaining bulge. Another problem with trying to lose fat around your waist is that our bodies want to keep it, not just as a source of energy but also to protect our vital internal organs from cold weather. Fat is an excellent insulator so our bodies first eliminates all fat from our appendages such as arms, legs and face before using the fat that is stored around our torsos.

All of this can be very frustrating and cause the person to give up and go back to eating the same as they did prior to losing the fat which of course causes them to gain all of the fat back again. This is why any form of dietary change has to involve lifestyle and mental changes as well. It has to go all the way to the core of your being and not just be a superficial attempt at improving your figure.

It is a fact that all healthy diets no matter of what type will produce dramatic fat loss. What you have to understand is that it is not a steady-state process and that your strategy needs to change along with your current metabolic situation. My advice to people who want to improve their physiques is that they will gain more muscle and loose more fat by reading about the process than actually going to a gym and working out. What I mean of course is that you have to be smarter and better educated than your body on this subject, and your body, my friend, has a million year head start on you!

19 KETOGENIC RECIPES

Here are some standard Keto recipes to get you started. They are mostly desserts and all of them taste like their high carb relatives but eating them will cause you to loose fat. For more recipes go to www.ruled.me or any of the other keto recipe websites.

Avocado Mint Chocolate Chunk Ice Cream

I make 4 kilos at a time and freeze it in small containers.

Ingredients

Mint flavoring to taste (preferably natural powdered mint)

Vanilla flavoring to taste (preferably natural powdered vanilla)

2 ripe avocados

1-cup coconut milk

Half-cup heavy cream

Half-cup of unsweetened baker's chocolate cut into 1/4" chunks. (approximate size)

Sweeten to taste with powdered stevia

Preparation

1. Cut the avocados in half and scoop their insides into a bowl.

2. Add the cup of coconut milk, half cup of heavy cream and 2 tsp. Vanilla.

3. Blend this mixture together until smooth and creamy.

4. Blend the chocolate chunks and stevia into the avocado mixture.

5. Place in the freezer for about 10 hours to freeze.

6. Remove from Freezer prior to eating so that it can soften.

Keto Maple Syrup

Ingredients

3/4 Cup of water

1 Tbsp. of unsalted butter

2 1/4 tsp. Coconut Oil

2 tsp. maple extract

1/2 tsp. vanilla Extract

1/4 tsp. xanthan gum to thicken

Sweeten to taste with stevia

Preparation

1. Mix your butter, coconut oil, and xanthan gum together in a microwave safe container.

2. Microwave the mixture for 40-50 seconds.

3. Mix microwaved oils and water together.

4. Add vanilla and maple extract and powdered stevia to taste. Thin with water if needed.

5. Microwave for 40-60 seconds, stir, and let cool.

Keto Pancakes

Ingredients

4 Tbsp. Heavy Cream

4 Tbsps. of flax seed

2 Eggs

2 Tbsps. Peanut Butter

2 Tbsps. Keto Maple Syrup

1/2 tsp. baking powder

1 Tbsp. Butter

Preparation

1. Mix Peanut Butter, Maple Syrup and eggs together.

2. Add the 4 Tbsp. Heavy Cream.

3. Mix in the flax seed and baking powder.

4. Grease a skillet with butter at medium heat.

5. Cook the pancakes until the tops bubble then flip over. Cook for an additional 1-2 minutes.

Strawberry Preserves

Ingredients

16 oz. Fresh Strawberries

Powdered Stevia

5 tbsp. Chia Seeds

Preparation

1. Slice the strawberries into small pieces.

2. Place strawberries in a pan over medium heat.

3. Let it simmer for about 5 minutes, until the juice has thickened slightly.

4. Add the chia seeds and stir for about 2 minutes. Remove from heat and let cool. The Chia Seeds produce a coating of gel when in contact with liquid. They will thicken the jam and are very good for you as well.

Strawberry Milk Shake

Ingredients

1/2 cup Coconut Milk

1/2 cup Heavy Cream

4 tbsps. of the keto strawberry jam

2 tbsps. coconut oil

Preparation

Place the ingredients in a blender. Blend to the consistency you want. Other types of fruit can be used for variety.

Keto Chocolate Chip Cookies (2g Net carbs per cookie)

Ingredients

1-1/2 cups Almond Flour

5 tbsp. powdered egg whites

3 tbsp. Coconut Flour

3 tbsp. Psyllium Husk

10 tbsp. Unsalted Butter

3 tsp. Vanilla Extract

1 tsp. Baking Powder

2 Eggs

1 bar Unsweetened Chocolate diced into small pieces.

Powdered Stevia.

Preparation

1. Mix dry ingredients together.

2. Beat warm butter with an electric mixer for 2 minutes.

3. Add the egg and vanilla to the butter and beat until combined.

4. Sift the dry ingredients over the wet ones and mix well.

5. Mix the chocolate chips into dough. Divide the dough into 22 equal pieces.

6. Roll dough into balls, place on a cookie sheet and flatten.

7. Preheat oven to 350F and Bake for 15 minutes.

Ketogenic BBQ pulled chicken breast

Ingredients

2 boneless skinless chicken breasts.

3 cups tomato sauce

6 finely chopped garlic cloves

1 finely chopped onion

9 tablespoons cider vinegar

3 tablespoons Worcestershire sauce

3 teaspoons paprika

2 teaspoons freshly ground black pepper

2 teaspoons chili powder

1 teaspoon celery seeds

Add Stevia to taste

Preparation

1. Mix ingredients, except chicken, in a small pot over medium heat until they come to a boil.

2. Add Stevia and vinegar for sweet sour taste.

3. Add the boneless skinless chicken breasts and let simmer about an hour until very tender.

4. Use a couple of forks to shred the chicken breasts.

Thai Sweet and Sour Cucumber and Onion Salad

Ingredients

4 Large Cucumbers, unpeeled and sliced

2 Red Onions, sliced

2 Cup White Vinegar

1 Cup water

Sweeten to taste with Powdered Stevia

Preparation

1. Prepare the cucumbers and onions. Place them in a Tupperware container that has a secure lid.

2. Add the other ingredients.

3. Add more vinegar to increase the sour flavor, more Stevia to increase the sweetness or water to reduce both. Let it marinate for a few hours in the refrigerator and serve. If you let it marinate long enough the cucumber slices turn into pickles. I then add dill and clove to make dill pickles.

ABOUT THE AUTHOR

I'm a 66-year-old 5'8" 180lb. bodybuilder. During the last year I have had 4 different facelift procedures done in Thailand, a massive heart attack while under sedation followed by 2.5 hours of CPR and a one-week coma. A month later my weakened heart went into congestive failure so severe that I could not walk 15 feet without being out of breath. Along the way I went through a divorce after being married for 30 years and 3 basal cell carcinomas. I should have died many times over but having decided that there was no viable up side to that strategy I did my research and found cures for all of my afflictions, well...except for the divorce, that one just keeps on giving.

Only 5% of CPR recipients survive longer than 30 minutes. That must put me in the 1% group. Only 50% of extended coma victims survive. 40% of all congestive heart failure patients die within the first year. I currently walk a mile to the gym every other day, lift the same weights as prior to my CHF and then walk back to my apartment. Additionally I walk a couple of more miles each day to shop or visit friends. All of this is in Arequipa, Peru at an altitude of 7,500' where there is 17% less oxygen per breath. I'm a serial survivor who should have died many times over and I have been trying to analyze and quantify the why of it ever since.